'The Fattened Lions on the
Educational Odyssey'

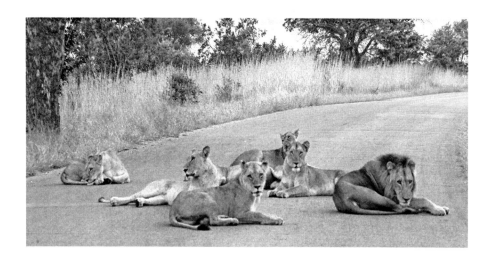

'The Fattened Lions on the Educational Odyssey'

The Autobiography of Hope Gangata
(A case for raising aspirations and widening access to higher education)

Hope Gangata

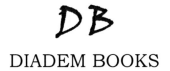

DIADEM BOOKS

The Fattened Lions on the Educational Odyssey

All Rights Reserved. Copyright © 2012 Hope Gangata

Published by Diadem Books
Distribution coordination by Spiderwize

Diadem Books
16 Lethen View
Tullibody
Alloa
FK10 2GE
Scotland UK

www.diadembooks.com

ISBN: 978-1-908026-47-7

"To be, or not to be: that is the question"
From *Hamlet* by William Shakespeare

Table of Contents

Acknowledgements

I HUMBLY ADMIT Lendy Thobejane (Nee Lendy Swartbooi) made a critical impact on the development of this book. The initial impetus to pen my autobiographical memoirs occurred after I proofread a working draft of her own autobiography entitled *Innocent Little Faces*, whilst I was in Cape Town. The book portrayed how she grew up in a gripping disadvantaged mixed race community and matriculated at Ravensmead High School in Cape Town in 2002 to become a university graduate in theatre performance. The book draft was *"a testimonial struggle that I have been through in order to finally pursue higher education at one of Africa's top higher institutions. This book is especially for young adults to learn from and relate to."*

She always had her community youth at heart. Even during the throes of her university learning and examinations, Lendy continued to teach drama to children in her very own neighbourhood against all odds, attract a team of volunteers and cobble together funding from a plethora of sources.[1]

And now six years and innumerable sleepless nights later, *baiedankie* (thank you) for the lasting impression you made on me.

---

[1] http://www.uct.ac.za/print/mondaypaper/archives/?id=6289 and
http://152.111.1.87/argief/berigte/dieburger/2007/08/01/KS/14,15/ks-showbiz-nebo-459.html

It was quite touching to have a massive gust of support and encouragement behind my back. Help in writing the book has come from all angles that 'were so great a cloud of witnesses' to my life and autobiography book. I have been exceptionally blessed to have close friends from all over the world that immensely helped me review the book, in Europe, Africa, North America and here in Norfolk. My first school contemporaries helped with verifying the primary school chapter, each wave of contemporaries having helped with the respective chapters. They reminded me of some glaring omissions of events and corrected some facts I was now hazy on. I honestly wonder how the book would have stood on its two feet were it not for the thoughtful contributions I received. Credit should be given to modern electronic technology, such as email and Facebook, for enabling rapid communication with the reviewers. Thank you copies of the book with personal messages are working through the postal hoops to them. Following is the list of friends who gave editorial assistance:

Alaine Mukene (England)

Allison Lamont (England)

Allison Lee (USA)

Anita Williamson (England)

Antony Chipazi (South Africa)

Benjamin Gangata (Zimbabwe)

Bernice Gangata (Zimbabwe)

Bethany Smith (England)

Blessing Dumbura (Zimbabwe)

Bonani Dube (South Africa)

Boykie Makay (Zimbabwe)

Brent Meredith (England)

Brian Mapani (South Africa)

Bruce Gangata (Zimbabwe)

Byron Manuhwa (Zimbabwe)

Chris Warton (South Africa)

Christopher Columbus Gangata (Zimbabwe)

Claire Brockwell (England)

Cleyson Mupfiga (South Africa)

Dave Chikosi (USA)

Edgar Shoniwa (South Africa)

Emily Bowora (South Africa)

Estelle Gangata (Zimbabwe)

Esther Gangata (Zimbabwe)

Felix Kagura (South Africa)

Gemma Apps (England)

Heather Landwiski (USA)

Helen Risebro (England)

John Brown (USA)

Lazarus Kuonza (Uganda)

Lex Loizides (South Africa)

Lisa-rose Moller (Scotland)

Lydia Munyi (Kenya)

Magret Moyo (Zimbabwe)

Maphios Siamuchembu (Zim)

Mazengenya Pedzisai (Zimbabwe)

Mehluli Sibanda (Saudi Arabia)

Mellisa Ilboudo (Sierra Leone)

Micheal Paketh (Zimbabwe)

Mitchell Bontle (South Africa)

Mpendulo Magutshwa (Zimbabwe)

Nicola Robinson (England)

Nompilo Mtunzi (Australia)

Ntsako Khosa (South Africa)

Oana Fodor (Romania)

Phatheka Ntaba (South Africa)

Preeti Lall Durowoju (India)

Princess Akol (South Africa)

Robert Ndou (South Africa)

Samuel Maviyani (Namibia)

Sandile Pazvakavambwa (Namibia)

Sarah Edwards (England)

Sarah Nhamo (England)

Simba Takuva (South Africa)

Tafazdwa Mungwadzi (Zimbabwe)

Tapiwa Kwambane (England)

Terry Sikweza (South Africa)

Thandeka Ngcongo (South Africa)

Tsitsi Gono (Bermuda)

Tsepiso Nyopa (Lesotho)

Uapa Pazvakavambwa (Namibia)

Valentine Marume (Zimbabwe)

Vyvienne M'kumbuzi (Rwanda)

Zandile Ramma (South Africa)

A special thank you goes to all the people of whom I have mentioned by name in the book, who have allowed me to share part of their private lives with the public for the sake of raising aspirations among young people.

The first book publisher I approached, Diadem Books, under the editorship of Charles Muller, a former Professor of English, was delighted to publish the book after the submission of just the first two written chapters. The publisher has been very helpful in formatting and checking the English of the book.

My mother visited me in England for four months in the middle of 2011 and it was her first maiden trip abroad. She bravely started learning how to use a computer and to familiarise herself with the layout of the keyboard, I gave her various handwritten pages of the book to type. During the first few days she took the whole day to type five sentences or so, whilst battling to use the computer mouse and Microsoft Word software! Towards the end of her stay she could easily type ten pages or so. I was amazed – within a space of two months after she was back in Zimbabwe, she had typed 16 000 words of the first three chapters of her very own autobiography, starting in the 1950's, on her laptop!

I wanted to show my dad a copy of the book, but there were obstacles. He is unfamiliar with computers and was living on the other side of the country to anyone who could take it to him. My sister, Estelle, printed the entire book and took five days of her time to travel 200 miles from Bulawayo to Mwenenzi to give him the copy. She waited three days for my dad to read the entire book and came back to Bulawayo to email me his comments. That was sweet of you, Estelle.

My desire was to have seven lions representing the metaphorical fattened lions lying on a road for the book's front cover. I was spoilt for choice after I obtained permission from several photographers. I am grateful for the photograph taken by Mr Arno Meintjes from Nelspuit in South Africa, which I finally settled for.

I have been very humbled by the strong support I have received for the book from various organisations and institutions. I have received offers to give talks to schools, public talks and interviews from radios, even before the book had gone to press. The talks have given me the opportunity to fine tune a 40-minutes PowerPoint presentation summary of the book using photographs of my youth not included in the book. Please feel free to contact me if you are keen on me giving a talk to a group of youths, or would like me to give your class a presentation of growing up on the other side of the world, and a break from the usual schoolwork. I hope to build on the initial thrust of the book towards aspirations of children from non-professional families by communicating with the public using the www.youthaspirations.co.uk website.

Last but not the least, I was thrilled and felt honoured to receive the support and advice from Emeritus Professor Susan Standring, the Editor-in-Chief of the 39th and 40th editions of *Gray's Anatomy: The Anatomical Basis of Clinical Practice, Expert Consult,* on making the book flow better. She took time off from her busy schedule to read the whole book of my journey into the anatomy world and wrote the foreword for the book.

Heartfelt deep thanks to everyone who was associated with the writing and sharing of ideas connected with the book, including those not mentioned in the above acknowledgements.

Hope

Foreword

'If you do not think about your future you cannot have one…'
(Galsworthy, 1867)

AROUND THE WORLD, tens of thousands of young people cannot think constructively about their future because they lack the appropriate knowledge and advice that others, living in more fortunate circumstances and with access to advice and mentoring, take for granted. In his autobiography, Hope Gangata takes us on a long and fascinating journey from his childhood in Zimbabwe to a lectureship in East Anglia, UK. He describes the many challenges he has faced and overcome so successfully, sharing his experiences while studying and working in the post-apartheid nations of Zimbabwe and South Africa and travelling in Central and Southern Africa, the Middle East and Europe. What shines out from the pages are Hope's growing self-belief and steely determination to achieve his goals, tempered by a thoughtfulness for others and a desire to share his experiences with the next generation, all underpinned by a strongly held Christian belief.

I know from my long association with a widening access to medicine programme that many students who come onto the programme will have had very little, if any, guidance from their school or their home about planning their future lives. Ignorant of what might be possible, far too many have low self-esteem and little confidence in their abilities, believing that all they can expect from life is a dead end job or unemployment – not surprisingly, they fail to appreciate the value of education and self-discipline because nobody has demonstrated that these things are important. Hope addresses these shortcomings in his book. He challenges his readers to raise their aspirations and to think positively about their future, in other words... *If you think about your future you can have one.....*

Susan Standring PhD., DSc., FKC., FRCS (Hon)

Emeritus Professor of Anatomy, King's College London
Editor-in-Chief of the 39th and 40th Editions of *Gray's Anatomy*
President of the Anatomical Society of Great Britain 2008-2011

Chapter 1

Infancy in Bulawayo

A ND THERE WERE NO LIONS THEN…
The 'rain scent' is utterly unforgettable. For there were only two seasons in the Zimbabwean city of Bulawayo–rather dry, mild winters and wet summers. The winter temperatures barely fell below ten degrees centigrade during the day and jerseys were for the frail. The summer heat dried whatever was left of the savannah after the winter, and the torrential rains came halfway during the summer season. The mornings were classically sky blue without a cloud in sight, especially around 10 a.m. The rains almost invariably came during the midday heat, at lunchtime, and scuppered plans of pupils of going home after school. The rains were earth shattering, customarily punctuated by streaks and flashes of lightning and claps of thunder, all within a space of twenty minutes or so. You would be soaked to the bone if you spent any longer than a minute in that rain. It rained cats and dogs.

Bulawayo, in spite of these rains, was an incredibly dusty city and is only rivalled by Pretoria, in South Africa, on the 'city dustiness' index. It was the fusion of the torrential rain and the hot dusty earth that generated the 'rain scent', a combination of rain vapour from the hot ground and the newly freed soil and earth chemicals. It was unforgettable, especially when associated with the wriggling of my tiny bare feet into the recently created warm mud puddles! After the rain, by 4 p.m., the sky would regain its impassive blue composure once again, as if nothing had happened.

The massive street was as straight as a pencil and was laid out on land as flat as a tabletop. I inquisitively took my four-year-old body to the edge of the street and lo, I could see the streetlights for over two miles! That street, Main Street, could accommodate two cars abreast travelling in one direction and two other cars abreast going in the opposite direction whilst still allowing four rows of cars to park face to face.

"The streets were built to accommodate two rows of horse carriages travelling in opposite directions," an old man once murmured.

The sides of the tarred street were officially brought to an end by a concrete hard shoulder. After the kerb, there were the unmistakably straight rows of mature Jacaranda trees, providing a shaded walking space that reached the fences of the houses, just like Pretoria, as I was to experience later. How glorious the purple Jacaranda trees were at the start of the rainy season, creating a velvety carpet that was so scrumptious against our bare chubby feet! This Main Street was almost eighty years old in the 1980's and was flanked by six other similar majestic roads on either side. The last street on the western side of the city centre was called Lobengula Street, after the name of the last king of the Ndebele kingdom, Lobengula. The street was the 'Berlin Wall' of the city and frontline limit for Blacks before Independence. Going across Lobengula Street required the magical apartheid 'pass cards' that proved that one had a job as a gardener or maid, that permitted entry into the leafy and well maintained enclave of this once White controlled sanctuary. The shops beyond Lobengula Street were more of the English blend like Woolworth Stores or Smith's Jewellery. Not too many people were keen on shopping beyond Lobengula Street either, as the marked prices were much stiffer.

That was Bulawayo, the second largest city in Zimbabwe. Of all the twenty odd cities I have visited across the world, the city planning of Bulawayo beats them all. A young city with hardly any building older than 100 years, Bulawayo allowed the city planners to build from a blank sheet. Older cities, like London, Nairobi and Casablanca, suffer the handicap of having to work around existing infrastructures, the end product being a hybrid of the older city and the unfulfilled dreams of the city planners. Bulawayo had huge open areas all over the city: parks, open land, low density houses in the north and east, high density areas in the west and a vibrant industrial area in the south. The prevailing winds always blew the polluted industrial air towards the high density townships. Car drivers from the townships had the calculated misfortune of facing the sun in the morning while going to work and also when returning home. The fellows from the 'posh' side of town never had to shield their eyes from the glare of the sun when going to work or returning home.

Bulawayo had a fascinating history of different groups conquering it and is one of the important linguistic nerve centres for one of the Nguni languages, Ndebele. The Nguni languages are a very peculiar group of languages and are the only languages in the world with 'clicks'. The 'clicks' resemble the sound of pebbles falling on water. A lovely simple video description of how to vocalise the different 'clicks' sounds can be found on the Youtube website.[2] The late Miriam Makeba made a beautiful, traditional song famous, a song heavily laden with 'clicks'. [3]

In 1789, a man was born who changed the face of the Nguni languages. His name was Shaka. Shaka was intent on empire building the small Zulu tribe into a formidable kingdom at a high human cost. Using a combination of newly invented and highly

---

[2] http://www.youtube.com/watch?v=31zzMb3U0iY&feature=related
[3] http://www.youtube.com/watch?v=6aNZ8qwKDrE&feature=related

effective military techniques, he conquered and assimilated the smaller tribes with a mix of intimidation and diplomacy. The empire building spewed out splinters of the Nguni speaking tribes that were escaping the assimilation and the human fleeing was called the 'Great Scattering' (Mfecane). The Ngwane tribe fled to Swaziland. Three splinters of the Ndwandwe tribe defeated by Shaka fled to Mozambique, Malawi and as far as Tanzania, close to the Equator.[4] They ran a distance of 3000 miles through thick bush with no roads, teaming with hordes of wild animals. It was for good reason. Shaka was well known for sending long-distance regiments to pursue escaping tribes.

One of Shaka's army generals, Mzilikazi, felt he had come of age and defied Shaka. He broke off with the Khumalo clan in 1821 and trekked north slowly for 19 years from South Africa until he and his followers arrived in Bulawayo in Zimbabwe in 1840. Mzilikazi plagiarised the name of the capital city of Shaka and also named his capital city Bulawayo. He displaced the poorly organised Shona tribes living in Bulawayo. After the death of Mzilikazi in 1868, his son Lobengula ascended the throne, but was forced to flee in 1893 when British colonial forces took control of Bulawayo under Cecil John Rhodes. The army of Lobengula besieged the colonial settlers for some months but never regained control of their home despite several bloody battles that inflicted heavy casualties on Bulawayo's new residents. Under the British colonialists, Bulawayo prospered and had its wide streets planned out and built. Bulawayo was declared a city in 1943. Later, after an eight year civil war, Zimbabwe won Independence from Britain and created more equitable public services.

---

[4]See map on page 6.

I was born and had my childhood in Bulawayo, which was dominated by a Nguni language. I later travelled to Zululand, Swaziland, Malawi and Tanzania and I should say it is rather comforting to know that all the people of the Nguni languages could understand my spoken Ndebele well! My family lived in the residential side of the central business district of Bulawayo at No 3A Main Street. It was a humongous house with five bedrooms, two corridors, three lounges and three verandas. At the back of the house were all sorts of fruit trees. There were about twelve mango trees that bore a lot of fruit but the Indian landlord stripped the trees bare to make their annual supply of mango chutney. It was a bit unfair because we watered the trees and paid dearly in high water bills. I always dreaded being left alone in the house, especially at night as it was so spooky, but fortunately there were always tenants taking up the excess capacity of the house. Televisions were not yet common in the early 1980s and at night the creakiness of the vast wooden floors freaked me out. This was pretty normal, as I was only four years old. The living room was spacious and had a full complement of sofas enveloped with a light brown artificial leather cloth fabric. A centre coffee table completed the set. I have a family picture when I was in that room and it can be seen on the photograph sections of 'The educational odyssey - the autobiography of Hope Gangata' Facebook group or the www.youthaspirations.co.uk websites.

The time arrived to attend pre-school and my parents chose the Jewish Hebrew Nursery school, about six blocks away. We were one of the first groups of Black children to be accepted there. The school was the preserve of Jewish children before Independence in Zimbabwe. It was a nice tidy school that had a broken down cabin of a truck for us to play in. We would turn the steering wheel this way and that way, pretending to be truck drivers. Running in and out of the truck was fun for us. Friday mornings at the pre-school were my favourite times. We were each given the ingredients to make a candy boat and we would take it home afterwards.

It was at about this time that my twin younger sisters were born. It was quite a surprise to have twin siblings. They were so identical that it took my mother a year to tell them apart! The only clue she had was that one of them had a natural earring hole on the surface of the lobe of one ear.

Map of Bulawayo

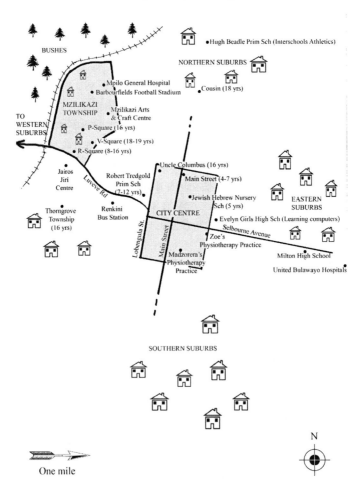

Chapter 2

Fantastic Primary Schooling

THERE WAS A CHARMING PRIMARY SCHOOL that shared its fence with Lobengula Street called Robert Tredgold School. Apartheid had ended only four years earlier in 1980 and this school had been previously earmarked and demarcated for the Indian community, and did not try to hide its strong Indian infusion. Everyone could now attend the school. However, some girl pupils still wore Indian saris over and above the school uniform, as did some of the female teachers. The school grounds were meticulously kept green and were separated from the main school by a comprehensively fenced permanent stream we called the 'donga'. The uniform was a well-conceived impressive cream two-piece safari suit. The short-sleeved shirts had a top pocket for pencils and two large pockets lower down in the front of the tummy, big enough for any bun. The shirts were complemented by nicely trimmed smart shorts with two front pockets and one at the back. How I loved these uniforms. The brown boxed school bags, fashioned like bulky briefcases carried by other pupils a couple of years before I started my first grade, were beyond description. And that was where I had got a primary school place.

On my first day at Robert Tredgold Primary School in January 1984, I was brought in by my mother. The morning schedule of registration events ended up allocating me to Mrs Noah's class, the 1A Class. After the mothers left, it proved to be a traumatic experience for some of my newly found classmates who cried uncontrollably for their mums, especially those who had not

7

attended pre-school before. I had been fortunate to have been to kindergarten and was used to mum leaving me at school, unlike some of the others. It was as if they had been dumped at a bus station to join a bus with no familiar face on it or being left on another planet alone. The classroom was respectably clean and well resourced. Every necessary commercial chart for learning was in our class and every child had an abacus for counting during maths sessions.

Lobengula Street, and not the Main Street, was the heartbeat of the city. It was the first and last street the natives could possibly use in town. Embedded in it was a massive bus station, a fruit and vegetable market with over 200 stalls, numerous stores, a large Indian Kravashe Temple hall and the Robert Tredgold and Mckeurtan Primary Schools. The presence of hundreds of vendors almost swamped the streets, and congestive street heart attacks occurred when lethal traffic accidents took place and everyone drew closer to come and see. The Lobengula bus station pumped public buses to the rest of the residential suburbs and townships, especially the high density Western suburbs. I have yet to see a contender in terms of size from the other world cities I have visited. This made the area the most dangerous in terms of traffic and we were religiously told by our teachers to always turn our necks this way and that way before endeavouring to cross Lobengula Street. Cars, trucks and people moved quicker during rush hours. Surprisingly, the businesses were dominated by the Indian community. Shops like Vasanjee Trading Store and Naik Clothing were the norm on Lobengula Street.

When I was in Grade 1 and 2 at Robert Tredgold School, the Grade 7 pupils were huge and a large number of them shaved regularly. The primary school first football team was like a men's team and was called the Open Age group team, which had no age restriction. To preserve the peace at the school, the teachers made them prefects. Being held by the collar by one of these prefects of renown made one immediately put one's tail between one's legs. The reason was that the 'comrades' had sacrificed their education to fight the war of Independence and they had to start from where they had left off. By the time we were in Grade 7 in 1990, almost all the Grade Sevens were normal twelve-year-olds.

Indeed, Robert Tredgold Primary School was an incredibly diverse school with interesting official catchment areas. The catchment areas included the Black township of Mzilikazi, a Coloured township of Thorngrove, and the houses to the immediate east of Lobengula Street, which had a significant portion of the residences of the part of town where Indians and Europeans lived. At one point a young boy from the Gujarati Province in India appeared at my desk with an exceptionally thick Gujarati childlike accent. It so transpired that I was the only one who could pronounce his name in one go during that year. His name was 'Nirow Mite Scomari Pareth' and the four words were blended together to sound like one word! There were five classes for each grade, with the brighter kids going to the A classes and the weaker pupils to the D and E classes. We had swimming lessons at the school pool once every two weeks.

During my second grade, my parents applied for a divorce, which took three years of legal wrangling to conclude. In the meantime, I moved from the city centre to live with my maternal grandma in Mzilikazi township. Mzilikazi had been the social epicentre and one of the oldest townships for Blacks for decades. If it had a website, it would boast of the following.[5] On one side it had the busiest road in Bulawayo, Luveve Road, which had one of the worst carnage vehicle rates in the city, especially at the traffic lights near the Mzilikazi Petrol Garage. Luveve Road was 'the street' that threaded through most of the Black townships to the

---

[5]See map on page 6

city centre. The second largest football stadium in the country (Barbourfields Stadium) was at the opposite end, close to the colossal Mpilo Central Referral Hospital where I was born. The stadium gates were normally opened in the last ten minutes of matches to relieve exit congestion. That was when the whole troop of my generation would enter for free and see the glamour of the football stars for a few minutes before the final whistle. Mpopoma Train Station, which breathed out trains to every corner of the country, was nearby. The oldest and most crowded township in town, Makokoba township, was the only thing separating Mzilikazi from the city centre. It had a market with the widest selection of traditional medicine, concoctions and herbs in the whole country. Things like leopard claws, monkey hides and some drinkable fungus suspension were traded openly. The fungi suspensions were later banned by the Government after the fungi grew in the stomach of someone who drank it. Whole tobacco leaves, that were probably the remnant of exported tobacco and were about two feet long, were openly sold in the front yards of many houses for a token amount.

There was a well-known Jairos Jiri Centre for disabled people in Mzilikazi website. Many years before I was born, there was a man called Jairos Jiri who lived a few houses from our house in Mzilikazi. Although Jairos was of a poor upbringing, he gave all he could to the poor. He even boxed so as to take the match winnings to feed the disabled in a patient, non-judgmental and tolerant way. He was a big guy with the softest of hearts. He set up the centre in a painstaking way over decades and eventually housed over 500 disabled persons. State disability allowances were an exotic term in the colonial days. It was a time of 'each man for himself and God for us all'. For income, curios were crafted and the Jairos Jiri musical band frequently hit the top of the national charts, led by a blind rapper Paul Matavire. Upon the death of Jairos Jiri in 1982, he was declared a National Hero and even dignitaries such as Mugabe took time off their schedule to attend his funeral in the Shona speaking countryside. Jairos Jiri is the Zimbabwean equivalent and quintessence of Mother Theresa. I do not know the extent to which the presence of a large community of disabled persons influenced my later choice of physiotherapy, but perhaps in some way it prepared me.

There was a community centre containing the Mzilikazi Arts and Crafts Centre, the MacDonald Hall, a library and a green park in the heart of Mzilikazi Township. A school leaver's recreational centre offered young people training in drama and ballet dancing. I was an active member of the library and the annual subscription was a mere 25 cents a year for kids. I remember whilst in primary school reading books from the library such as *Robinson Crusoe, Gulliver's Travels, The Swiss Family Robinson, Ivanhoe, The Legend of Sleepy Hollow* and *Rip Van Winkle*. Other books were the *Three Musketeers, David Copperfield, The Coral Island, Tom Brown's Schooldays, Treasure Island* and *The Adventures of Huckleberry Finn*. There was a dearth of English novels with local context. The impressive Mzilikazi Arts and Crafts Centre groomed painters, who worked using either pencil or oil on canvas techniques, and produced a vast array of pottery-making equipment. It was here that I shook hands with the then Prime Minister Robert Mugabe when he was having a political rally at the MacDonald Hall with its 1500 seating capacity. He got out of his car and was passing by the crowds and shaking hands with people on either side with a cheerful smile. I was hesitant to wash my right hand that evening. The second largest long-distance bus station (Renkini Bus Station) and a permanent river stream were the other geographical landmarks of Mzilikazi. Such a backdrop set the scene for an action-packed childhood.

It was an exceptionally fashionable trend for each boy in the neighbourhood to have at least two self-made gadgets: a toy wire car and a catapult. The wire cars were about the size of two loaves of bread, placed side by side, and were controlled in a standing or walking stance with a long extended steering wire rod. The wires were untangled from discarded or derelict fences, and in some really daring cases, from standing fences. Each wire was straightened out the 'stone age way', by gently grinding the wire between two stones with flat surfaces. One surface was a smaller hand-held stone and the other surface was a massive stone or concrete slab. A strong three-dimensional eye was essential, otherwise the end product would be awkward and asymmetrical. As a natural progression of the evolving competition to make better and sleeker designs and our increasing maturity and dexterity, almost every conceivable car or truck was synthesised. Some trucks had up to three detachable trailers and strips of bicycle tyres were stitched onto the wire tyres to give the wire cars a professional touch.

Mzilikazi was surrounded on one side by miles of bush sprinkled with shrubs laden with seasonal berries and perennial birds. There were catapults galore and they were crafted from 'V'-shaped tree branches, while the elastic portions were made from strips of car tyre tubes. Bird hunting was conducted in many of the bushes surrounding Mzilikazi and brown sparrows and pigeons were the common birds caught. My accuracy was not very good and the first time that I finally landed a bird on the ground was a very memorable one. I had half a second to emerge from next to a shrub, turn around to look to the right and aim squarely at the chest of a small red bird with a literally deadly blow. The hunting was so enticing that it continued among the houses and whenever windows were smashed, responsibility was blatantly denied. Occasionally the sparrows were caught alive with bin top traps. Some bird grub was placed under a bin top, which was about 70 cm in diameter, and a stick made the bin top stand on one side. The stick was remotely controlled by a twenty-metre string that would be pulled once birds went under the bin top and collapsed it.

By the time I was ten years old, each child at school in the 1980's was entitled to a free 200ml carton of milk, which was decorated with designs of African wild animals. The presence of milk was becoming a status symbol. The milk was then sold and was banned a while later, when it transpired that it was only the children of the wealthy who were getting the milk, due to the incessant price hikes. All our exercise books were provided by the government and had large inscriptions of 'Ministry of Education' on it; aaaah, the good old days!

There was a young girl whom I crucified mathematically in Grade 4. By the end of Grade 2, I knew my multiplication tables inside out, and could work out any grocery change mentally. The girl was hopeless in maths but always had these glorious sandwiches filled with avocadoes, stewy mincemeat, bacon filling, you name it. I always had a 'communist lunch box' of plain bread and margarine, and cream soda or raspberry drink for washing down my small throat. We shared a desk and the mutual envy was soon levelled up. We created a secret Maths-Sandwich stock exchange which actively traded readymade maths answers and readymade sandwiches. She was only interested in the answers and not how they were worked out. At the end of that year, she was demoted to a B class. I was not surprised! I personally lost out too. The following year, I was sadly relegated back to the 'communist lunch box'.

'Hope, Hope, Hope…' and 'Hope, Hope, Hope…' were the chants that the hundreds of schoolmates sang with all their might. Most were standing and jumping and the weather was at its best in April. I was concentrating on the race battle and could barely appreciate the encouragement. This was one of the highlights of the year. It was the annual school sports day and I was one of the best 100-meters sprinters for my age group, of children born in 1978. Those were the days of Carl Lewis, and he really inspired me. I seemed to come up as number one among my schoolmates but never made an impression when I competed with other schools at the Interschools Competitions held at Hugh Beadle Primary School in Northend suburb. This was where the entire primary schools from the eastern, northern and southern suburbs, or the rather well off part, of Bulawayo competed in athletics. Only the competitors went to Hugh Beadle School. Each school had a section cordoned off with a large name label on it. Both the school and regional school athletics events were brilliantly organised. The transport arrangements, presence of the teachers, name tags, refreshments, meals, good and fair umpiring of races and trophy presentations were all above par.

The best part of my primary school days was the afternoons at home. We religiously played football on an open dusty area at the square of our neighbourhood almost every afternoon of the year from 2 to 7p.m., save for Christmas and New Year's holidays. On school holidays, it could be football from morning to sunset. Our football passions were inflamed by the presence of the second largest football stadium in the country about half a mile away. The township was one of the national football hotspots that generated a steady stream of national football players like Peter Ndlovu, Mercedes 'Rambo' Sibanda and Tito Paketh. Tito Paketh lived about ten houses from my home and often created small prizes for the winning lads. The football 'thingy thingy' from my township sort of rubbed off on me and I was not surprised to be named the 'Top Goal Scorer in the School' when I was in Grade 5. For my efforts I was given a pair of size five 'takkies', some canvas shoe trainers, which proved too tight for my feet. Those were the days when I was growing fast like a weed.

Boy oh boy, I had tonnes of adventures when I was a boy. On one of my school holidays around the age of twelve, I decided to start a small business venture. The venture was obviously illegal, feasible and required no tremendous financial acumen. The plot was elegantly simple and involved buying unfrozen small sachets of drinks, that we called 'superkools' ('lollypops'), sold in packs of ten for 45 cents and selling them frozen at ten cents per sachet to make $1, to long-distance travellers at a 'Renkini' bus terminus. The 'Renkini' bus terminus was second largest in the country only to the infamous 'Mbare' bus terminus in the capital city and was a mere one-mile away. The wholesaler of the 'superkools' was located in the vicinity of the bus station. We had a large modern fridge that could squeeze and freeze a decent six packets overnight and on the selling day, I could fit four packets into my schoolbag and two into the box I would use to sell them in. Old newspapers were a critical component of the good insulation system and a leak from one of the 'superkools' would mess up my schoolbag. Renkini was one of the busiest areas in the city and had buses to every corner of the country. Travellers carried luggage, small livestock, furniture, large farming implements, 50kg packets of cement and colossal bags of agricultural produce. There was aggressive touting for travellers by the bus drivers, bus conductors and unofficial conductors called 'mawindi'. The 'mawindi' were remunerated off the books with kickbacks from the official conductor.

The appearance of a traveller holding travel bags would elicit a 'Renkini reflex'. It simultaneously involved the driver revving and moving the bus slowly forward, half the 'mawindis' grabbing the bags to place them onto of the bus and the other half banging the sides of the bus creating a frenzy that would paralyse the decision-making process of the would-be passenger. Deception was rife! The official bus conductor would then majestically appear on the scene and calmly and reassuring pull out the ticket book. After the issue of the bus ticket, the driver would reverse back and switch off the engine to save his fuel and the 'mawindis' would go back to chatting behind the bus, while the new passenger began to be concerned at what time the bus would eventually leave the bus station. The lack of the

'Renkinireflex' was no auditory respite; the place was incredibly noisy and the buses would play their radios at full blast playing tunes from Michael Jackson, UB40 or Bob Marley and the Wailers, to the accompaniment of vendors shouting bargain prices for their wares.

One in ten people there was probably a professional mugger called 'matsolas', who would pickpocket, swindle the gullible out of their hard earned money or simply take home the luggage during the 'Renkini reflex' commotion instead of taking the luggage to the top of the bus. It was smoothly done in such a way that you would be too ashamed to explain the ordeal of how you lost your luggage when you got home. The presence of the second largest police station (Rose Camp Police Station) ten metres from Renkini, forty times larger than Renkini, was rather embarrassing, given the mayhem and terror caused by 'matsolas' at Renkini.

It was in this pulsating and vibrant bus station that the twelve-year-old Hope launched his financial escapade, as the embodiment of senior partner and salesperson. The khaki-wearing policemen had their work cut out – catching the 'matsolas' or vendors red handed and creating order at the bus station. The difficult part was to catch them during the illegal activity and the policemen would be unknowingly chatting with the vendors (with the merchandise hidden) and the 'matsolas'. So whenever I was sorting out the change for a customer, my other eye would be scanning behind my back for the men wearing khaki. Once a vendor was caught, the police simply confiscated the merchandise or fined you, whichever was less. I dreaded having my stock confiscated and always kept an eye open.

The financial motivation for my clandestine adventure has confounded me to this very day. On a good day I made a profit of at least $2 per day, which was deposited into my Post Office savings bank account on my way back home. The Post Office was about 300 yards from my dwelling. At the end of the five-week school holiday, I had a healthy bank balance of $45, which I later dipped into during the school term. I had thrown caution to the winds and ignored the policemen. My hard work under no supervision, in spite of the lurking policemen, just to save money for absolutely no good reason or financial need, still baffles me to this day. There was always more than enough food at home, my clothing was in good shape and my school fees were always paid. I will shake the hand of a twelve-year-old chap who can do the same while under no financial pressure.

At the nearby shops 'Emachipsini shops', where we bought our morning bread and milk for our 'communist lunch boxes', real fried chips and fish were sold. The potatoes had a distinctive strong flavour, which was attributed to the right potato species and rich red soils of the Zimbabwean farms, the likes of which I have not seen on all the continents. Just the smell alone of chips, as one neared the shops, was enough to launch one into a soul searching mode and question why one was so poor as not to be able to gratify a simple appetite. Man! Those chips were always a couple of financial brackets above us. Once in a blue moon I bought the chips and washed them down with 'an orange tarino' carbonated soft drink. The bottle had an ironically twisted shape that tempted everyone to untwist it at one point or another. I would walk in the opposite direction from home while eating them, lest I should meet any of my envious close friends – or even worse, having the news reach home that Hope was enjoying a scrumptious and lip-smacking meal with the inevitable conclusion: "No wonder he has no appetite for evening 'sadza nemavegi'!" 'Sadza nemavegi' was a notorious Zimbabwean budget staple diet of cooked corn flour (corn meal) and green spinach-looking vegetables. Our usual consolation was 'amacrumbs', the crispy remains of fried chips, which were sold for a tenth of the normal price of chips. The downside was that the supply of 'amacrumbs' was unpredictable and they were generated once every four hours or so. The presence of a customer who had been waiting over an hour for them could easily scuttle any 'amacrumbs' episode. That meant one could not leave home with the certainty of buying 'amacrumbs' at the shops.

The hair-do for boys in Zimbabwe then was a dreadfully no-win situation. Girls escaped the ordeal by braiding their hair into cornrows. It is unthinkable that a certain school in London has banned cornrows![6] I think they should have organised a national pressure group of some sort to address our concerns. The cost of keeping up appearances was just too high. There were three realistic options: keeping an afro, uneven trimming of the hair or an absolutely bald head called a 'zuda'. Keeping an afro over half an inch in height was gruesome to comb and the jaws of the hair usually did not allow a comb to trespass through the terrain. Even after a spirited and tearful hair pulling exercise with the comb, the hair would look like it had never been combed by the time one arrived at school, and meant that the school prefects would brandish yet another comb for you to start to comb again. Trimming the hair was the best option. In those days, there were no electric hair trimmers and normal scissors were used. The evenness of the hair was atrocious and looked like a swarm of praying mantes had had a field day on your hair. The hair looked even and much better after a week or so of growth, but in the meantime, the neighbourhood would be getting top notch rib entertainment. The sight tickled your friends to death. The 'zuda' was the worst option. It was done with a hand-held razor and any unpredicted head movements would result in a small cut. Generous portions of 'Vaseline' were usually applied and ensured a literal 'top sparkle', which attracted slaps from

---

[6]http://www.bbc.co.uk/news/uk-england-london-13350098

schoolmates. School hats usually did the trick of hiding either the uneven hair trimming or the 'zudas', but once the too-good-to-be-true news wriggled out, one had to defend one's hat from being pulled off for a week or so at all costs.

The country Rhodesia (former name of Zimbabwe) had just come to the end of an apartheid racial political system in 1980. The recently born Zimbabwe was led by Robert Mugabe, as the power-wielding Prime Minister, while President Canaan Banana was the ceremonial President. Zimbabwe was the pride of all the African nations and frequently newspapers and magazines would tell us how high we were ranked on the international happiness, health or literacy indexes. There were expatriates galore ranging from medically trained staff and teachers to highly skilled people helping to rebuild the country, although some were simply attracted by the Zimbabwean dollar. It was the mightiest on the continent and one Zimbabwean dollar cost two United States dollars or one and half British pounds. Those were the days when picking up any lost coins on the streets translated into pocketfuls of sweets. Everyone was 'nicey nicey' to us – even the Queen of England did not miss the opportunity to knight Mugabe, as Knight Commander of the Bath, one of only a couple of foreigners to receive it. It was very rare for any country to require a visa from a Zimbabwean passport holder. The strength of the Zimbabwean economy was legendary.

The origins of the strength could be traced back to Prime Minister Ian Smith, who unilaterally declared independence from the British Crown in 1965. In retaliation, sanctions were applied to Rhodesia and Smith set out to bust the sanctions by crafting a well-rounded economy, so as not to depend on outside production. He really tried his best, although the cream of the economy was ring fenced for people of European descent while frugal provisions were made available for the rest of the 'others'. By the time Mugabe was given the country in 1980, Zimbabwe had the most diversified economy in Africa. Mugabe created greater educational and health opportunities for the native Black population. Zimbabwe was one of the few African countries with its own national airline. It was the second African country to have a broadcasting station, after Nigeria and ahead of South Africa. Zimbabwe had its own medical school at the University of Zimbabwe that trained medical doctors to consultant level. The literacy rates and immunisation rates were the highest in Africa. Hospital treatment was totally free, even for having surgical operations and was modelled on the National Health Service (NHS) of the United Kingdom. A highly educated population and the presence of the University of Zimbabwe ensured that tertiary industries such as consultancy and banking thrived and were in top-notch condition.

Commuter buses criss-crossed the city every five or ten minutes like clockwork, just like the London buses, while we paid a mere six cents fare as children. The agricultural sector was the best in Southern Africa and exported throughout the region. The weather temperature hovered from 10 to 32 degrees Celsius and encouraged the planting of crops throughout the year. Hunger was unheard of, and no one died of hunger related causes. The milkman would leave bottles of milk on the doorsteps of houses in the morning. Stray dogs and cats did not touch the milk, as they always had enough food. Even the newspaper man left the morning newspaper on the doorstep and went his way. It was pointless to have a brilliant agricultural system that grew the best tomatoes but could not transport them to town because of bad roads. Therefore roads were made throughout the land and almost every farm had a land phone line. Tourism was well marketed and hordes of foreign currency loaded faces were more than happy to go for safaris in the national parks and pay homage to Victoria Falls. The falls are the widest in the world and are over 1.7 km wide and the water drops for 110 meters.

In Zimbabwe's hey-day, most world star musicians held live concerts in the two major cities. Even Bob Marley made a song passionately entitled 'Zimbabwe!', which he first sung in one of our stadiums (Rufaro Stadium). Mining was the pride of the London and American investors and gold bullions with a vast compendium of metals being extracted from the Great Dyke, the southern end of the Great African Rift Valley. The sporting teams were not doing too badly either. The women's hockey team had won a gold medal at the 1980 Olympics and cricket, rugby and football had a very strong junior school policy. Street kids were an unfamiliar and foreign concept. Almost every house in the cities had piped water, sewage systems and state subsidised electricity. We had an electric train commissioned in 1983 from Gweru to Harare, a rare feat by then for an African country.

Every other African nationality was looked down upon by Zimbabweans. The Mozambicans had been in a deplorable state of civil war for decades, Malawians were looking for any menial jobs in the farms and Zambians were having an unbelievably high inflation and were literally buying bread with thousands of 'kwachas', the Zambian currency. The Batswana from Botswana were the only high chinned nationals and were well off; they paid any amount for schooling in Zimbabwe and came in large numbers. The educational system in Botswana was exceptionally weak, such that, to enter the army or police force, one just needed a primary school leaving certificate. There was nothing equivalent to A-levels in Botswana.

We never ever met any Black South Africans, and now I realise that it was very strange and weird not to have seen any. The first time that I saw a Black South African was when I went to South Africa at the age of 28, although we were neighbouring countries. Had I met one I would have grilled him with many questions, on what he was doing here, what he ate, and so on. Black South Africans were an unknown and mysterious people in

Zimbabwe. All we knew was that there was a nasty racial segregation going on there on the other side of the Limpopo River. The smallest to the greatest of us knew that Nelson Mandela had been locked up and the keys had been thrown far away. Songs like '*Something inside so strong*' by British singer-songwriter, Labi Siffre, correctly conveyed the emotions going on at the time.[7] Mandela was finally released in 1990 during my final year of primary school, and Zimbabwe declared it to be a public holiday.

The teachers during my primary school years managed to beautifully submerge the school curriculum into our playful characters without us noticing it. I was up-to-date for my age in my reading and mathematics abilities, without having to study in any way for the tests. I was progressing so well that I was a serious contender for the top positions in class. My first ever class prize was at the end year examinations in my Grade 3. I became a villain the day following being told I was getting the prize, after I broke one of the classroom windowpanes unintentionally.

"Hope was too excited," snorted my classmates.

My second and last prize in primary school came when I achieved the first position in the Grade 7 class, which was actually a tie with a tall girl called 'Nokuthula'.

Our Grade 7 class was under the firm and no frills tutelage of a tough short Indian lady by the name of Mrs Pashotum. She had a sort of a permanent pimple on the knob of her nose and frequently shrugged one of her shoulders to align her sari dress. Those who dared her by not pitching up in class with a duly completed homework triggered her to say, "You will be soon

---

[7] http://www.youtube.com/watch?v=n-i9CUAAHN0

sitting on the top of the dustbins on the street corners." She did not miss the opportunity to add, "Chewing chewing-gum like a goat!" if you were caught red-handed chewing chewing-gum.

She confiscated any tennis balls the pupils were playing with near the classrooms and wrote RTS on them, the abbreviations of the Robert Tredgold School.

Her bark was worse than her bite. Unlike most of the other teachers, she never beat or spanked anyone, but her admonishing and reprimands touched you to the core. Most of her former students only realised later how invaluable her strict regime was. It was with profound sadness that I learnt that she had passed away a few years ago in 2006 due to a brain tumour.

It hit me like a ton of bricks how much I had grown over the seven primary school years. It was now time to move on and I was ready to start secondary school.

Chapter 3

Competitive Secondary Schooling

MY OLDER BROTHER AND COUSIN were attending Milton High School, and the most logical and logistically easier thing to do, was to attend the same school. Prior to 1980, the school had been reserved for White boys only and so had excellent infrastructure. On the entrance to the school hall, there were wooden engravings of 'Old Miltonians' who had died for Britain during World War One and Two. There were lists of names of former Head boys and captains of the first rugby, cricket, hockey and athletics teams of the school on decorative panels hanging on the inside of the school hall. The pupils were called by their surnames and hardly anyone knew another pupil's first name.

On the first day at Milton High School in 1991, I was allocated to the 1:3 class based on my Grade 7 results. The first number of a class represented the Form and the second number the particular class among the academically screened ten classes per Form. The Grade 7 results were graded from One to Nine, with a Grade One being a top grade and Grade Nine being the worst grade. The pass mark was a Six grade and above. I had achieved a Grade One in Mathematics, a Grade One in English, a Grade Two in General Science and had a Grade Five for Ndebele. The Ndebele had undermined my overall aggregate, even though it was way better than my mother tongue Shona. We were required to write a Form 1 screening test, about a week after we started, which was composed of Mathematics and English only. As a consequence of the entrance test, I was moved up to a 1:2 class, which was quite a cordial class. I did not create any enemies or very close friends either. At the end of the year I was number two in class and was promoted to the 1:1 class which was then called the 2:1 class, because a new year had just started. The 2:1 class was in a league of its own.

The students in the 2:1 class were nerds of the highest order. Even the jokes they cracked were more book based, like the 'van der Merwe' jokes and the 'knock knock who's there' jokes. That was very unlike the jokes in the 1:2 class, which were more from everyday life. Most of the students in the 2:1 class were from the eastern and northern (the more affluent) parts of the city, while most of the students in 2:2 class were from the poorer western section of the city. Only a handful of the students in the 2:1 class played any sports at all and I will not count chess as a sport. They all claimed not to have read nor prepared for any of the tests, only to find that usually five of the guys had 100% in a mathematics test. I never saw one of them staying after school to read or study. They all disappeared and went home. I had no study room at home. I simply read my school books on the sofa or cleared the kitchen table if I wanted to draw graphs for maths. My aunt would easily find house chores for us to do if we were doing nothing. We jumped into the nearest book to pretend we were reading when we saw her coming into the house.

Fortunately, all the pupils at Milton High were given personal copies of the standard textbooks covering all their subjects. Some subjects had more than one textbook, like English Literature, Geography and History. Losing a school textbook meant that your examination results were withheld until a new replacement book was bought. Everyone understood the textbook rule perfectly. Although getting these books was a blessing, as my parents were not the textbook buying type, it was a curse in a way. The distance from home to school was a solid eight miles.

Carrying my burgeoning 'communist school satchel' of at least twelve pounds in the sweltering October heat, being jam-packed with at least ten textbooks, ensured sweat-soaked shoulders on our boyish body frames. The school was joined to the city by a massive Selbourne Avenue Road, which was as straight as a pencil for a good mile. The length of the linear road made walking such a bore for it appeared as if we were not making any progress while walking. Fortunately, the trees on the pavements made the walking bearable.

I quickly developed a good sense of my strengths and weaknesses and hence developed a game plan. I was first-rate in mathematics and sciences and feeble in Art, French and Ndebele. Whenever the class marks were given out for the latter subjects, I would cross my fingers and hope that I had avoided the bottom ten. My target for mathematics and sciences were to be in the top five in class. Mathematics was quite straightforward and whenever the teacher announced a date for a chapter test, that was the time I stopped reading for it. I would only check my formulas the night before the test. At the end of the first term, I was number 17 in a class of 35 pupils – I had feared the worst. I was exasperated by pupils who performed exceptionally well across all the subjects. I was normally pleased to get percentages in the 70's or 80's for mathematics and sciences, only to find some guys had mathematics and sciences marks in the higher 90's. I was even more horrified to learn that the same chaps who had 90's in mathematics and sciences, also had 90's in Art, French and Ndebele! I thought it was by fluke until after about four school terms, with the mark profile still unchanged, I gave up pursuing them. In all the three years I was with that class, the only time I was in the top ten in that class was when I was number seven on one of the terms.

We had three terms in a year. In the first and third term, we had to wear a summer uniform, and a winter uniform during the second term. The blazers were relatively pricey for the average parent and the decision to buy a blazer was made even dicier by the rapid growth of the arms of the 13 to 16-year-old boys. When my dad bought me a blazer, one could hardly see my fingertips. By the time I was in Form 4, the sleeves of my blazer ended halfway between my wrist and elbow. I had to shrug my shoulders to make the sleeves of the blazers move closer to the wrist. I was lucky! The parents of the other pupils could not afford one and the boys usually wore one of their father's jackets that was nearest to navy blue. These blazers were called 'bachis' and had varying designs and an unpredictable number of buttons, unlike the recommended school blazer which had two front buttons. In winter, any students wearing 'bachis' caught by the prefects were noted for detention or punishment. Some were made public examples during the school assembly, much to the heavy ridicule by the rest of the school assembly. The prefects had considerable authority and they were allowed to cane and punish any offenders who crossed the school rules.

Milton High School firmly believed in giving glory to outstanding pupils. Anyone who was granted permission to purchase 'an academic tie' by the Headmaster was considered one of the sharpest tools in the shed. They had to have had five straight A grades at O-level on one certificate paper. The ties were grey in colour, unlike those for the rest of the school which were navy blue. Those students who excelled in sport had their names gloriously announced during school assembly. Their names and usually their chubby faces were also published in the school magazine and they became a seasonal celebrity. Their real bonus was being given permission to purchase 'a grey colours blazer', a blazer which was any colour as long it was a dull grey. It was very easy to spot a 'colours blazer' from a quarter of a mile away, as it was distinct from our navy blue school blazers. The 'colours blazer' was the easiest way to charm your way through the neighbouring high schools.

When I was in Form 2, the Minister of Education, Fay Chung, a Zimbabwean born lady of Chinese origin, abolished all the 'other funny national subjects' taken at the end of Form 2, like French and Art. The move galvanised my strengths, eliminated my weaknesses, and streamlined my efficiency. She resigned the following year and all the 'other funny subjects' came back, but only after I had crossed the Form 2 examination bridge. Fay Chung had previously taught in underprivileged Black schools in Gweru and had orchestrated teacher training and curriculum development in Zimbabwe's pro-independence refugee camps in Tanzania and Mozambique through the 70's.

The Zimbabwean Government had a communist policy in the 1980's, with politicians referring to each other as 'Comrade so and so' on TV. The governing body was the Politburo. They really meant business and were dead serious when they shouted the 'Health for All' and 'Education for All' slogans. For example, only 5% of the Black Africans in Zimbabwe in 1980 had access to basic education, but by 1993, 95% of Zimbabweans of the school-going ages had completed primary school, which was conducted in English. The donor community supported the post-war recovery wholeheartedly. But the accounting books were not balancing up and so they approached the International Monetary Fund (IMF) and the World Bank for some fresh loans. The moneylenders prescribed a capitalist medication, which cut across the communist grain, and the Government obviously refused to take it. The Government hobbled on for the last half of the 1980's without any outside help and that ensured a stagnant economy. Stifling investment policies and conditions limited foreign investment. Manufacturing entered stalemate and under capacity because they could not acquire foreign currency to buy spares and import raw materials. I witnessed the dramatic changes in the welfare of some pupils whose parents were made redundant in the factories.

In those days, companies could only acquire or sell foreign currency from the Government controlled Reserve Bank of Zimbabwe and externalising foreign currency was a grave sin. Some precious wealth from the state coffers were also used to send Zimbabwean troops to Mozambique to help their Government fight the RENAMO, who were bandits financed by South Africa. By 1990, it was clear that an economic Plan B was now needed. In July 1991, the Finance Minister, Bernard Chidzero, launched a World Bank backed Economic Structural Adjustment Programme (ESAP). ESAP entailed lifting of the communist price controls, a 40% currency devaluation, a relaxation of import controls, reducing government expenditures by retrenching 25% of the civil servants and cutting parastatal losses. In a nutshell, ESAP meant taking on a capitalist pinch and making the country more open and market-driven. Six months later, when I was 14 years of age in Form 2, the worst drought in more than a century hit the subcontinent, and ESAP was limping. We thought then that it was the worst ever situation.

The national economic sneezing trickled down to my level. As teenagers, we had started to assert ourselves and develop our own opinions on things and would give good reasons for doing certain things. That did not help matters at home and our needs drifted towards the fancier direction. Sony Walkmans, movie ticket money, lunch money, more presentable clothing and more pocket money than we had in primary school were sought after. A pair of new simple 'Bata' shoes would have sent us over the moon in primary but now the more elegant 'Grasshopper' shoes were more appropriate. Otherwise the whole 2:1 class would be unleashed into a laughing frenzy by the news that Hope has new 'Bata' shoes! We had reached a point where we would not be seen wearing a pair of shorts without a pocket! We had come of age. We lived in the poorer section of town but went to school in the more well off part and so we were exposed to finer clothing. Each and every day, we had to pass the chic restaurants in town only to go home to 'sadza nemavegi'. In the process, we harassed and besieged our appetites and nostrils with the fine cuisine of the restaurants and arrived home with dislocated and misaligned appetites.

Catching two buses to school was no longer a financial option. ESAP was growing roots and it was being bellowed time and time again on national TV that everyone 'has to tighten their belts'. Walking or cycling to work or school was becoming popular as the economy began to grip. I had always longed for a bicycle but it was always beyond my fiscal depth. When I was 14 years of age, news reached my ears that there was a slightly older guy selling his 'bike'. The size 24-inch 'bike' had spent a myriad of seasons in an open air shed. The 'bike' had mere shreds of tyres on its wheels, had lost about half of its ball bearings, and needed pedal replacement. It was going for a whopping $20! After analysing the tantalising bargain, I informed the guy that I was going to source the money. I managed to source the money, with half of it from my mum. In little over a month, I had replaced the missing parts, sand papered and resprayed it with a silver green colour. I paid for the City Council Bicycle Tax disc and attached it to the handlebars. (Yes, even bicycles were taxed!)

I removed the brakes, mounted a perry brake system and a pedal gear cog with 52 teeth, the largest available in the land. The addition of a rear cog of 12 teeth ensured brutish and adrenaline-pumped speeds. At that age and being one of the boys with the fastest growing bones south of the Equator, I could not achieve enough knee clearance on the bicycle handlebars on the size 24-inch bicycle. To alleviate the tight squeeze, I fused two seat poles one on top of each other, so as to increase the height of the seat and welded motorcycle handlebars onto it for knee clearance while turning. It looked cool and had a flair of designer uniqueness. The 'bike' was rebranded and was renamed

'Quagga', after the half zebra that had become extinct from the plains of Southern Africa, just some 100 years earlier. I loved my 'quagga' and kept it in almost perfect condition always.

In the first term of Form 3 in 1993, we started preparing for O-level examinations over a two-year period. Only the first three of the ten classes could study sciences and the first two classes were given the option of choosing an additional subject of either French, Ndebele and Additional Mathematics. I disliked linguistic gymnastics of any sort. I chose the Additional Mathematics subject, which assumed knowledge of the ordinary O-level Mathematics subject, and was half of an A-level subject. As 15-year-olds, we learnt intricate jargon like 'the product rule of differentiation, integrating by parts' and became conversant with advanced trigonomical formulae in Additional Mathematics. It conjured up an air of prestige in so far as were known as 'the Additional guys' by our fellow O-level classmates.

English literature was compulsory and the poetry book gave me grief. For a poem of a mere 30 words, we were asked to write three pages about the author's feelings towards trees on one of the poems for 25 marks. For the next term, we would be asked a very similar question like 'whether the author's feelings towards trees was real' on a fresh three pages. I always ran out of linguistic steam and inspiration after writing half a page of that poetry stuff. Nothing was typed in those days. Oh, how I hated the class readings of *Great Expectations* by Charles Dickens! We had to read *Romeo and Juliet* and the book tormented me. It took me one solid hour to read one page, as the book was written in old English prose. After every second word or so, I had to look at the explanatory notes and dictionary. By the time I had referred to the dictionary or explanatory notes five times, I would have forgotten what the first sentence was all about.

My reading consolation was a book entitled *Animal Farm*. It was a mere 100 pages written in simple English. The final discarding of a horse called Boxer, a huge horse with the strength of two horses put together, broke the hearts of our entire class. He had worked exceptionally hard in building the windmill twice over and was a key figure during the Battle of the Cowshed and the Battle of the Windmill, which were in defence of the farm. However, Boxer was sold alive, when he was poorly, to be boiled down at the knackers for a bottle of whisky for the ruling class of the pigs.

Towards the middle of the second term in 1993, the Bulawayo section of the Ministry of Education received a consignment of ten computers from some donors. Two high schools were selected to pioneer an O-level subject of Computer Science and they chose ten boys from Milton High School and ten girls from Evelyn High School. The computers were housed at Evelyn High School.[8] The boys with the ten highest marks from the 4:1 class in Physics and Chemistry were selected and I was eighth on the list. We went on Wednesdays at 2 p.m. and this was some two years before Windows 95. Those computers were devilish and so encrypted to use. In simple words, one had to master a programming language before being able to use them. Once switched on, a minus sign on the 14-inch black and white computer screens would blink continuously. If you dared to type in a word that was not in the vocabulary of the programming language, the computer wrote 'SYNTAX ERROR' and reverted to the blinking minus sign again! The programme that can be installed on Windows computers is available from the BBC website[9] for those keen to have a go at it. Those latest computers had a 'whopping' 16 MB of hard drive and 32 KB of RAM! Information was stored on floppy discs the size of an A5 exercise

[8] See map on page 6
[9] http://www.bbcbasic.co.uk/bbcbasic.html

book. The 'Dot Matrix' printers screeched noisily like a tree full of hundreds of small birds in the savannah sunset.

A triad of clandestine and surreptitious activities went on during lessons during the successive generations of the 2:1, 3:1 and 4:1 classes over the three years I was with the class. Somehow, I got caught up in the keeping of white rats. Our activities, which included keeping pet white rats, chess and gambling were carried out in the shadows of our school satchel while the teacher was busy teaching. These activities hardly happened in the other classes and the teachers did not even have the faintest idea of their existence. Over half the class kept pet white rats in the arm portion of their jerseys on any day at school, except on examination days, lest the invigilator saw some unexplainable fidgeting in the examination room. The food smells during the tea breaks aroused the curiosity of the rats and they would instantaneously poke their heads out of the sleeves of our jerseys or the top of the pockets, in order to assess the grub situation. The trick to give a rat a name to which it can respond, was to call the rat by that name while feeding it when it was young, preferably in the first three weeks. Fortunately the rats never chewed any papers of our homework books. The cuteness of the rats while eating a peanut with both hands was quite a memorable sight. We also had tiny magnetic chess boards that could be easily and quickly hidden underneath a school satchel if the teacher happened to walk across the classroom from the blackboard.

Towards the beginning of Form 4, we used to play hand gambles with 50 cent and one dollar coins, commonly referred to as 'ski' or 'chaputa'. A boy would hide a coin underneath his palm and the second boy would place his coin underneath the palm of the first boy. The second boy had to guess correctly which side the coin was facing to win it and would lose his coin if he failed. The practice came to a halt after we were caught and referred to the

Deputy Headmaster, Mr Manda, for caning. Mr Manda was the shortest among all the teachers, even among the female teachers. The only times he did not carry a long caning bamboo stick was when he was going to meetings or going home. Any sight of him by fellow pupils triggered a flight of refuge behind the classroom blocks. But on this sad occasion, there was no running away. The caning strokes were uninterrupted and landed hotly and evenly on our bottoms. Fortunately they did not tell our parents.

In Form 4, virtually all the students in the 4:1 class were convinced that the eight subjects we were being offered at school provided insufficient intellectual gymnastics. Thus most of us added two more subjects like General Science and Extended Science to our O-level Cambridge examination booking to make it ten subjects. The former was what everyone in the country wrote and the latter had equal portions of Chemistry, Biology and Physics. A few chaps registered for eleven subjects.

I lived in a house in R-Square in Mzilikazi that was a semi-detached bungalow with four large bedrooms. On swinging open the gates, which swung into opposite directions, one was immediately greeted with a single car parking space. The car park was for many years occupied by a Renault-8[10] car that belonged to Aunt Judith. The car was a bit weird because the engine was in the boot and had a storage space underneath the bonnet, which was for keeping excess luggage while driving. To the left of the car park was a large half an acre garden that was seasonally planted with corn, otherwise it had green leafy kale vegetables destined to make the grievous 'sadza nemavegi' dish.

Further afield the garden was a chicken run. Occasionally batches of five dozen one-day-old 'Irvine chicks' were bought

---

[10]http://en.wikipedia.org/wiki/Renault_8

and reared for two months and sold for a profit, with a few of the chickens augmenting our meat in the house. I had to bend over to enter the chicken run and grab a wing or leg, to start with, and then secure the chicken properly and tie the feet together, when a customer placed an order for a live chicken. At the end of two months, all the chickens had to be slaughtered and stored in Aunt Judith's large deep freezer, lest we ran into a loss with the cost of feeding chickens that were not gaining any weight.

Killing the chickens was not for the fainthearted. Both legs of a chicken were firmly held with the underneath of the left foot, while the two opened wings were fastened underneath the right foot. The left hand grasped the head of the chicken and the story was finished off with a knife in the right hand. After the chicken was dead, the whole body was dipped in piping hot boiling water for no longer than 20 seconds. The dipping allowed the plumage to be easily plucked off. The dipping for a shorter duration made the removal of the feathers impossible and a longer duration made the entire skin fall off. In one particular year, we had rabbits and it was an experience to see furless baby rabbits growing into adult rabbits, before they were also destined for the pot.

If one restarted from the car park and made a right turn, instead of a left turn to the garden, one walked on a concrete footpath to the main entrance of the house that was protected by burglar bars. The burglar bars opened into a small veranda that led to the lounge after passing through a pair of French glass doors. Grandma's bedroom opened into the small veranda while two other bedrooms were accessible from the lounge. The kitchen was the room further down the lounge and had the fourth bedroom opening into it. My older brother, Bryan, was given the fourth bedroom to give him tranquillity during his university studies. Aunt Judith used one of the two bedrooms and the other room was used by the three girls. The room allocation algorithm left me with the lounge to sleep in, for all the nine years I lived in R-Square. After a while, I got used to it.

In the spacious lounge we had two different sets of sofas. Each set had four pieces of a three-seater sofa, two-seater sofa and two single-seater sofas. The sofas faced a black and white television, which in time was upgraded to a colour television set. There was still room in the lounge for an eight-seater dining table. The TV broadcasting started at half four in the afternoon with children's programmes, such as 'Inspector Gadget' and 'Tom and Jerry' cartoons, while the most popular evening programs were 'Knight Rider' and 'Allo Allo'. My worst programme was some absolutely dull overrated American sitcom that popped up every Thursday evening without fail called 'Cheers'[11], which took great delight in filming the same faces around the same table weeks on end. It is a drama that must be avoided like the Bubonic plague and not worth the TV airtime slots that our one and only Zimbabwe Broadcasting Casting station[12] gave to it. Whenever it came up it triggered me to work on my homework.

Suddenly, things began to get rather messy and dark at home in R-Square in Mzilikazi from around late 1993. I lived with 'Gogo' (grandma), an aunt, an older brother, my two twin sisters and three other cousins. Four of the children were teenagers attending high school and the other three were still in primary school. Gogo usually spent part of the rainy season in the rural areas ploughing on her land inheritance in Headlands and in the winter selling embroidery stuff in Botswana or South Africa. I was in the outer circle of either my aunt or grandma. My relationship with my aunt slid terribly in the first few months of 1994, especially in the absence of grandma. I decided to move out and stay with my brother Bryan who lived in P-Square of Mzilikazi,

---

[11]http://en.wikipedia.org/wiki/Cheers
[12]http://www.zbc.co.zw/

who was in the middle of his BSc in Water Engineering degree at the National University of Science and Technology in Bulawayo. I stayed with him for a month or so and it did not work out, and so I returned to my grandma's place. It was a bad idea. After a week I went back to Bryan who had moved to Thorngrove township. This was not sustainable and by around April 1994, I went to sojourn with Uncle Columbus who lived near Lobengula Street in the city centre. That was my fourth packing and moving in a space of four months. There were consequences. The move decimated my day-to-day stress and halved my cycling distance to school. My dad hit the roof upon hearing I was staying with his younger brother. Nevertheless 1994 was an exceptionally special year for me, as that was the year I was writing my O-level examinations and so everyone's heads cooled off for the rest of the year.

My schoolwork had taken a turn for the worse and a ruthless and callous end of term school report signed by an exceptionally short Deputy Headmaster, Mr Manda, summed it up. He simply said that I 'would end up on the streets' at the rate I was working.

Uncle Columbus has always been my favourite uncle. Almost every other day after work, he would take Calvin, his first born son, and myself for a walk along Lobengula Street. He lived in town in Bertha Court on the next street to Lobengula Street, in the city centre. He never failed to buy us fruit like bananas and apples during the walks. He was known as the 'biscuit man' and kept a couple of carton boxes of Lobels biscuits in the house. The house was awash with biscuits for the late afternoon tea and, when he was in better moods, he gave the biscuits at any hour. Visits to his workplace were more magical! He was the chief electrician and a line manager at the Lobels Biscuit factory. Visitors allowed inside the factory would have the privilege of eating fresh moist biscuits to their hearts' content, straight from the conveyer belt.

My uncle had an unfailing love for an arcane vernacular State Radio 2 station. It beamed from a massive radio that was built into a wooden cabinet the size of the boot of a saloon car. The radio station had a quiz session that no one seemed to win called 'Jarzin man'. The programme was hosted by Admire Taderera and started with

"JARZIN, taka taka,
J-A-R-Z-I-N, (spelling it out loudly)
JARZIN, taka taka,
I am your money-man,
the Jarzin Man. Good morning"

The program was like a watch. The programme always started at 6:45 a.m. during the week. If you heard the program on radio during schooldays, then you knew you were going to be late for school. School started at 7:30 a.m. sharp and it took about 50 minutes to get there.

Bryan had been attending a new small church in early 1994 called Grace Christian Fellowship International Church (GCFIC) led by Pastor Dave Chikosi ('Pastor Dee'). I started attending GCFIC regularly, and, a few months later, I was born again. I was the third generation of Christians, the first being my grandma who lived in the suburb of Mzilikazi, Bulawayo.

My grandma attended a United Methodist Church in neighbouring Matshobane township that unashamedly conducted its service in Shona, despite being located in a predominantly Ndebele-speaking region. Church had been compulsory for years for the whole family. Granny always bolted and locked the house when she went to church, for there was no other option but to go with her.

At her church, worship songs were all from hymn books and the services were well attended by mainly elderly persons. I remember leaving the services with a respect and awe for God every Sunday and would be very careful what I said about the Deity. However, this attitude of reverence never lasted for very long. Sunday was the only day I took God seriously. The rest of the week was 'business as usual'. Church to me was all about a set of rules as a minimum qualification to avoid being thrown into hell.

The term 'born frees' in Zimbabwe referred to people who were born after the 1980 Declaration of Independence, and did not experience loss of human dignity on any level by reason of being an African. One thing that I had valued in my life was my liberty. I had preferred to live with grandma rather than my dad, because I had whole days to myself and was free to do as I pleased. Another Zimbabwean colloquial term that fitted me well was 'musaladi' (from the English 'salad'). Zimbabweans use this term to refer to people who have abandoned the traditional African diet in favour of Western foods. The South African equivalent is 'coconut'. This seemed an apt description of what I was evolving into as I grew up.

I was free from rural family pressures that lead many African peoples into ancestral worship. I am reliably told that I last visited my dad's rural village in Gokwe when I was one year old. I was also made to understand that the last time I had a trip to my mother's village in Chimanimani was when I was ten years old.[13] To date it has been over 24 years and I still have not visited any of the rural villages of my parents. And even though both my parents are Shona, my fluency in spoken Shona is average and my written Shona was atrocious and bordered on the verge of illiteracy. Up to this point in my life, I had never written a single sentence in

---

[13]See map on page 44

Shona. The reason for all this is because I grew up in Bulawayo, Matabeleland. We spoke Ndebele and I was fluent in it.

But even though this was Bulawayo, we only started learning Ndebele at school, about halfway during my Robert Tredgold Primary School days, and that may have contributed to my academic Ndebele being a practical stillborn. The parents of Indian and European pupils at the school had dug their heels against every pupil being taught Ndebele. When Ndebele was finally taught at the school, it was a watered down version of it called 'L2 Ndebele'. I was given the worst ever grade in the Form 2 Ndebele national examination and that was the last I saw of academic Ndebele. We spoke to each other in English as school friends, irrespective of whether we had met in the school grounds or kilometres away from the school. That was the default language setting among school-going children. I had a sprinkling of French when I was formally taught French at Milton for two years. Thus I was linguistically unhinged and had total liberty in a way. All the schools I had been at were culturally diverse and I was exposed to all sorts of things. I knew and cherished my liberty and my grandmother's church rules threw muck onto my glass.

God at Grace Christian Fellowship International Church was portrayed as Someone who was actively involved with our everyday living and not just chilling in heaven waiting for people to come for a Sunday church service. The congregation was so much younger and music livelier, like that of Ron Kenoly and Don Moen. No hymn books were used. Guitars, drums and keyboards were on the stage. God was the God of immediate miracles and not limited by time, space or the current state of affairs. Our righteousness was achieved through faith in Jesus who had died for our sins and presented us as clean before God. Our acceptableness by God was not through exemplary living or mighty deeds but simply by faith. I came to understand that guidance from God for us was meant to protect us. God's demand for holiness is partly because He wants to save us from the negative consequences of our sin.

He was presented as a God of not only eternal blessing but of 'blessings to the third and fourth generation'. Our actions, good and bad, have consequences that extend beyond the present. This is true even in the case of non-Christians. Their actions (illicit sex, drugs etc) have consequences that will affect generations after them. Academic social studies have established the very strong impression parents have on the social and economic standing of their children and grandchildren.

> *"The LORD, the LORD, the compassionate and gracious God, slow to anger, abounding in love and faithfulness, maintaining love to thousands, and forgiving wickedness, rebellion and sin. Yet he does not leave the guilty unpunished; he punishes the children and their children for the sin of the fathers to the third and fourth generation." Exodus 34:6-7*

We normally completed and sent applications for A-level places at the end of the second term. I had had enough of Bulawayo and made up my mind to go to a boarding school and move out of Bulawayo. Fletcher High School topped the list and required at least five red-hot A grades at O-level. I had purposed in my heart not to aim for 'bits and pieces'. Otherwise, you will always be envious of people who have gone for the full monty, i.e. gone for the full set. People applied for places before they sat for the examinations and I listed Milton High as backup. With each day moving towards the examination dates in December, my classmates would taunt me saying 'Fletcher Fletcher'.

The naked and pejorative second term report from the Deputy Headmaster reverberated in me like someone having a large legal case awaiting judgement. It was heavy stuff. The heaviness increased when I received the formal letters notifying me of the examination dates of the respective O-level subjects I registered for. I cobbled together a twelve-week reading schedule and started strategising my grades – the hard sciences such as Mathematics, Physics and Chemistry, Extended Science and General Science earmarked for A's. That was not enough, as the Fletcher High School place required 5 A's. The subjects that could generate B or C grades were Geography, Biology and English Language. History, English Literature and Additional Mathematics were frank borderline cases hinging on D grades and obtaining C grades would have appeased my conscience on any day. I had issues with them. I found History and English Literature to be too woolly and fuzzy for my liking and could not fathom how marks evaporated in my essays. With the rest of the subjects, I could easily follow where I lost marks and could make amendments to my learning deficits.

I went to stay with my dad after sitting the last O-level papers. He was always being shuffled among some small district offices around the country. This time he was in Kotwa town, in the hardcore Mashonaland region. It was a dusty growth point in the hot basin of the mighty Zambezi River near the Mozambican border. It had only two rows of shops on either side of the street. The only decent thing to do there was eating juicy sun-ripened mangoes, otherwise the heat swallowed up any other zeal. My spoken Shona had a permeating Ndebele accent and my Shona vocabulary was frugal and parsimonious, and occasionally floundered when some chap digressed into deep Shona.

My results came out in early 1995 and I was the last one to know. My mum had collected the results from the school and showed the whole neighbourhood and church chums and whoever was willing to listen. I travelled 700km to Bulawayo to see my results. I had obtained seven A's and three B's in Biology, English Literature and Additional Mathematics. I was ecstatic and remember squirming with excitement whenever I was alone in the bathroom. Fletcher High School was now game on after securing the 5 A's. I was convinced I had finally smashed into the top five in class with my results. The results of the other lads began to filter through like a veldt fire, despite the lack of us being able to meet at school. Cell phones and internet had not yet arrived in the country by 1995. The only currency that was used in comparing the class results were A grades, while C grades were not being detected on the 4:1 class results gossip radar. The top two had run away with ten straight A's, two chaps had 9 A's, four had eight A's and a whole half a dozen of us had settled for 7 A's. About 15 classmates had landed with five or six A's. The 4:1 class had been the only class that had pupils who had obtained 5 A's and above, some 25 out of 33 pupils. About 400 pupils of the school had written the O-level examinations that year.

The Fletcher offer letter duly arrived with the list of uniform and boarding item requirements, like single sheets, pyjamas and a lockable trunk. Dad wired the money to my uncle and I went with my aunt to look for bargains in Lobengula Street and off I went to Fletcher High School in March 1995.

Map of Zimbabwe

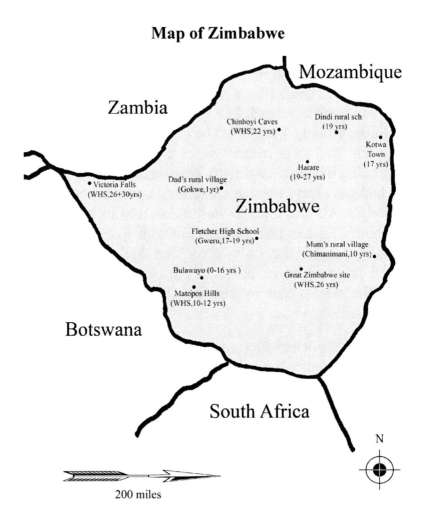

Mozambique

Zambia

Chinhoyi Caves
(WHS,22 yrs) •

Dindi rural sch
(19 yrs)
•

Kotwa
Town
(17 yrs)
•

Harare
(19-27 yrs)
•

• Victoria Falls
(WHS,26+30yrs)

Dad's rural village
(Gokwe,1yr)•

Zimbabwe

Fletcher High School
(Gweru,17-19 yrs)•

Mum's rural village
(Chimanimani,10 yrs)•

Bulawayo (0-16 yrs)
•

Great Zimbabwe site
(WHS,26 yrs)

Matopos Hills
(WHS,10-12 yrs)

Botswana

South Africa

N

200 miles

Chapter 4

Godly High Schooling

T HE 170 KM TRAVEL TO FLETCHER HIGH
SCHOOL in Gweru from Bulawayo passed through some
of the flattest and finest cattle rearing green lands, while my two
freshly loaded metal trunks were jolting on top of the rumbling
bus. The school was seated on a hill beside a small dam, Fletcher
Dam. Fletcher had been assigned for African students during the
colonial times and had a significantly weaker infrastructure than
Milton High. Everyone at the school, from the Headmaster to the
groundsmen, were Africans. The only exception was a Japanese
man who taught music and was on a Japanese sponsored
exchange programme. Having friends from a different race from
an early age is an important part of building racially tolerant
pupils. The lack of it creates distorted stereotypes, which are not
healthy. The bulk of the students at Fletcher had never been in
culturally diverse school settings all their lives.

Upon arrival at Fletcher High School, I was earmarked for the
recently cleaned Stanley Hostel, which was reserved for Form
5's (Year 12). Bruce Hostel had two dormitory wings attached to
a core building that housed the television room and the shower
rooms. The whole hostel was on ground level and lay on the
western edge of the school ground. Each dormitory wing was a
rather elongated large room with two neat rows of fifteen beds
and a complementary bedside drawer, upon which we placed our
steel trunks. Almost every school boarder in Zimbabwe had these
black steel trunks, which doubled as luggage bags and as security

safes. The trunks had padlocks to deter any wandering fingers that might pilfer the 'dog biscuits'. The 'dog biscuits' was the nickname we gave to the very popular uncreamed biscuits made by the Charhons Biscuit Factory and were sold in 2kg packages. The snacks of 'dog biscuits' and roasted peanuts came in handy when we burnt the midnight oil while studying.

After a couple of days we were asked to choose our A-level subjects. It was so crystal clear to my mind that I wanted to study mathematics, chemistry and a third science. I had a shifting sands dilemma of choosing between Biology and Physics. I had less passion and interest for physics but felt I would have excelled in it more because of my strength in mathematics and mechanics. Biology was quite the opposite and my keen interest in it mismatched with the grades I received during my O-level Biology course. The use of modern biological techniques to make commercial food, the molecular approaches of making vaccines and drugs and the intentional unlocking of high crop yields captivated my love for Biology. I followed my heart rather my mind and settled for Biology.

The school had nine classes of twenty students each: three humanity classes, two commercial class and four science classes. Two science classes had Mathematics, Chemistry and Biology whilst the other two science classes swapped the Biology for Physics. We had separate purpose-built laboratories for Biology. The laboratories were well equipped and had all the reagents and chemicals for Chemistry and Physics. We had both our teaching sessions and practicals for Chemistry and Physics in each respective laboratory. We were much more civil when we went for Biology and Chemistry classes, for it had enough chairs for all of us, unlike the survival of the fittest 'chair hunting' when we went for the Mathematics in the main teaching block.

There was a chronic chair deficit in the school by a factor of about 10%. The last few students to arrive in each class had to go 'chair hunting' in the vacant classrooms. Occasionally the parents association bought some chairs for the school but the natural breakage rate of the chairs always exceeded the arrival rate of new chairs. It never occurred to the school administration that the moving up and down of the chairs during the 'chair hunting' episodes contributed to the high breakage rate. The green lawns around the classrooms, which I had taken for granted at Robert Tredgold and Milton schools, were replaced with seasonally trimmed weeds. The sports fields needed an imagination on our part to appreciate their full extent. There was a very strong feeling that the school administrators had for ages been trying to run the school to the best of their capabilities with very limited funding. What an anti-climax it was!

There was a silver lining at the school. Fletcher High School had one of the strongest academic reputations in the entire country. Some 70% of A-level school leavers secured university places. In contrast, only a measly 10% of Miltonians went on to university and that was one of the reasons I left Milton. The school started with a better crop of students because they required 5 A grades at O-level. During the colonial times, only two schools were available for Africans to study A-levels – Fletcher and Goromonzi High Schools. The Europeans had access to over 100 A-level schools across the country. My father was a bitter man in terms of education. He had grown up in the rural areas of Gokwe and had a good primary school leaving certificate and had applied to Fletcher in 1969. The then Headmaster, Mr Alfred Knottenbelt, who had taught three generations at Fletcher and Goromonzi High Schools and had refused to raise and salute the colonial Rhodesian flag, set up a mischievous entrance criteria. A prospective student had to have stellar primary school certificate, submit a passport photo and pass an impromptu Intelligent Quotient test, which he conducted himself in his office. Having an 'unlooky' photo face meant a goodbye. My dad secured a place and progressed to finish his O-levels. In those days, no African could afford boarding fees for his or her child using their monthly wages only.

The foundation of the success of the education system in Zimbabwe can be easily traced to the illiterate generation of my dad's parents. They liquidated their cattle kraals to pay for educating their children – that was the value they attached to education, 'ma O revuro' (the O-levels as they pronounced it[14]). Such sacrifices are not common in other developing countries. My grandfather had a mammoth dilemma when my dad reached O-level. My dad's younger brother, uncle Israel, had passed his primary school leaving certificate with flying colours. However, the breeding rate of my grandfather's few cows could not cope with paying boarding fees for two sons. My grandfather decided that my dad could get a decent job with his O-levels and gave his other younger son an educational chance also. Uncle Israel secured a place at Fletcher High and went all the way to A-level, which he passed and proceeded to start a BSc in Metallurgy degree at the University of Zimbabwe in 1979. He was very active in student politics and was expelled in his second year and later passed away in 1997. That is why my dad was somewhat unhappy with his amputated educational career.

At the very core of the Zimbabwean education system lay schools such as Fletcher High. The best performing schools in the country had very basic school infrastructures. The schools with the best O-level and A-level results across the country were state or mission schools. Private expensive schools never made an impression on national academic school comparisons. The main university in the country, the University of Zimbabwe,

---

[14]The Shona language operates on only 23 letters of the alphabet and lacks the letter 'l', and so all the letter 'l's are replaced by letter 'r's.

hardly had any students from the top private schools such as Falcon College, Hillcrest High School or Peterhouse High School. Students from private schools were whisked away to study in South African universities, where entrance requirements were much lower but needed a larger financial muscle. People from outside Zimbabwe have found it hard to believe that Zimbabwean schools with their very basic infrastructures perform so well, while South Africa is following the American and British model, where the best academic results come from pupils from private expensive schools. The Zimbabwean approach is only possible if there is a strong societal and parental thrust for the pupils to exert themselves to the maximum and not rely on excessive personalised tutorship and other school frills.

I had come to understand fully that the responsibility of educating myself rested heavily on my shoulders and was not anyone else's liability. I had not had any of my parents coming to any of my 'parents consultation days', or had them buying a single textbook from a bookshop during my entire primary, secondary and high school days. My personal copies of all textbooks I had ever owned all my life were photocopies, with two pages being squashed onto A4 papers and stapled together. We blatantly and obviously took matters into our hands. During the last school holidays of 1996, just before the November A-levels holiday, my friends and I decided to have an August holiday study camp. There were five boys and three girls and none of us came from family backgrounds with professionals. It was dead easy to get permission to use one of the cottages that belonged to one of the teachers to use for accommodation because our group included the sitting school Head Boy and Head Girl. The cottages had no electricity and we used the school classrooms with electricity to study. Crazy enough, we used candles and torches for lighting and paraffin stoves for cooking in the cottages. Bulawayo was not an option and I had enough school stress to deal with already.

To get a good handle on Mathematics, one had to work ruthlessly through most of the problems in the *Pure Mathematics* textbook by Backhouse, *Concise Course in Advanced Level Statistics* by Crawshaw and Chambers and a mechanics book. We had obtained vast amounts of off-cut economy paper from 'Mambo Press Book Publishers' to use as scrap paper, that was charged by the kilogram. Moreover, I had Further Mathematics to contend with, cajoling with 'Crammer's Matrix Rule, De Moivre's complex numbers and forced harmonic motion', which required generous piles of paper. I was the only student who was studying A-level Further Mathematics at Fletcher High School. I had a different game plan for Biology. Over the course of the first term in 1996, I had painfully and tediously rewritten my own notes from three sources: my classroom notes, from the core textbook and from the notes of a friend, Simbarashe Takuva, who had finished the previous year. The new Biology notes amounted to two counter textbooks, which I covered in plastic. Chemistry was more straightforward and I compiled similar notes comparable to my Biology notes.

The Zimbabwean economy was now staggering in a drunken manner and the most visible symptom was the printing of the first large denomination note ($50 notes), while I was at Fletcher. It was a memorable moment finally to touch this new cool note. The highest note had been a $20 note since Independence in 1980. By 1996, a loaf of bread had rocketed to $5 despite being 25 cents at Independence in 1980. ESAP had obviously developed numerous economic mutations. Removing price controls caused consumer demand to shrink by 30% and fuelled inflation and consumer prices increased by 50% per year, from less than 15% per year throughout the 1980's. The inflation then caused real wages to go to their lowest levels in 30 years and also simultaneously reduced the real value of the Government budget. A double whammy of droughts in 1992 and 1995 created negative growth in those years. Street kids started appearing and slept on the city streets. An integral part of ESAP was to massively cut social spending and create cost recovery measures from consumers. The system of user fees erected tangible barricades for poorer fellows and hundreds of thousands of children were chased from schools due to non-payment of fees. The terms 'ESAP deaths' started appearing on patient notes written by doctors and nurses, indicating deaths were due to lack of money to pay for prescriptions, X-rays or to stay in hospital. The then Minister of Health, Dr Timothy Stamps, recognized that only 10% of Zimbabweans could afford health care on a cash basis. Thus the government launched the Social Development Fund (SDF) to assist poor households with school fees, health fees and food money subsidies. The first 'food riots' in living memory broke out in the city townships in 1993 due to runaway bread prices and a "bread boycott" lasted two weeks. Riot police had to guard our local shops in Mzilikazi for a number of weeks while carrying baton sticks. In May 1995, the IMF and the World Bank abandoned Zimbabwe after friction with Harare. Zimbabwe had 'one last chance' to realign the economy and ZIMPREST (Zimbabwe Programme for Economic and Social Transformation) was launched as the medicine to limit the signs and symptoms of ESAP in 1996.

There was church at the boarding school run by students under the banner of the Scripture Union. Just the thought of being the only child in a congregation full of elderly people was a serious church turn off. And so the Scripture Union at the school struck a chord and was interdenominational. We met every day of the weekday for about 35 minutes before supper in the school hall. Lives were changed, people gave their lives to Jesus and many pupils forsook their treacherous and perilous ways. We could not afford musical instruments, and even if they were there, there was a dearth of music-playing skills. The singing was augmented by a rapid clapping tradition. There were daily morning prayers about 30 minutes before breakfast. I was soon hooked onto the morning prayers and would go round the junior residence waking up the other mates for morning prayers. There was no service on Sundays, in order to allow people to attend their respective churches.

Towards the end of 1995 I was appointed to be part of the leadership committee. The leadership at Scripture Union had had a long, heart-breaking tradition of being 'academic insulators', stretching over ten odd years. They felt so strongly about the role of 'watching over' pupils who came to Scripture Union that the time management of their schoolwork dithered and was precarious. Only one Scripture Union Chairman or Vice Chairman had managed to be accepted into university in over six years. There were committee meetings on Friday evenings, where we prayed over newly arisen issues, planned for services and exhorted each other. These normally ended at midnight and that ruled out Fridays for studying. A minimum of three nights a week was spent on attending to pastoral issues among pupils. All mornings before breakfast were taken by the morning prayers and there were daily church services during the day every day except Sundays. I was doing four A-level subjects while everyone else in the school was taking three subjects. And so the time resource was really, really scarce!

The third and final school term started and all was set for the final A-level Cambridge examinations. With about two weeks to start the examinations I was hospitalised for about a month and missed the exams. Someone from home collected my belongings and my dad's 30-year unfinished A-level business remained unfinished. I did not say farewell to my classmates and friends from Fletcher High School.

I decided to finish my 'dad's 30 year unfinished A-level business' at Fletcher in the following year in January of 1997 and was set on sitting my examinations in June of that year. I had loved the school and it was like home. Upon my arrival back at the school the relations with all the people I knew had changed. I had to learn with guys who had been my junior and I was an outsider. My 1996 classmates were now wearing t-shirts that read 'Medical School of the University of Zimbabwe' or the 'Faculty of Engineering', while I was given the worst accommodation in the upstairs dormitory of Hanno hostel of Fletcher. My heart was almost broken when I saw an interview letter from Old Mutual. I had been short listed for an interview for a national Actuarial Science Scholarship to South Africa. The interview date had passed by two months. My Further Mathematics, good O-level results and my passing of the first round of National Mathematics Olympiad had strengthened my case. The National Mathematics Olympiad was extremely difficult and featured deceptively simple-looking pre-calculus mathematics problems that required untaught elegance and latitude and was written by A-level pupils. Who knows, I could have been a qualified actuary by now in 2012!

My dad was firmly against the idea of me going back to Fletcher and said he would not pay any of the school fees, although my education at Fletcher had not cost him anything. I had received my first ever scholarship from an organisation called Shamwari Dzevana VeZimbabwe (Friends of Children of Zimbabwe) that had funded my entire tuition, boarding and examination fees at Fletcher for the 1995 and 1996 years. Shamwari Dzevana VeZimbabwe never advertised and after I sent my application to an address in Harare, they sent a cheque to the school Headmaster. I have tried in vain to contact them to thank them for their belief in me. It has only recently hit me like a ton of bricks that the organisation was a charity set up by people who were from outside Zimbabwe; no wonder they were called 'Friends of the Children of Zimbabwe. My stepdad who had married my mum also said it was not his job to pay for my fees.

There were two things still needed to be paid, my A-level examination fees and tuition and boarding fees. I prioritised the examination fees and I did my rounds among my aunts and uncles. Thank God my aunt in Mzilikazi, Aunt Judith, chipped in with the entire $400 for the examination fees. Acquiring the money was only half the job needed to register for the exams. No school in Zimbabwe ever registered a pupil for A-level sciences who was not from their school and our school did not offer the examination in June. I was in hot water and time was running out. I had been playing cat and mouse games with the Headmaster, Mr Nyanhongo, that term. I had not paid a cent of the boarding or tuition fees well into the middle of the term. In desperation, I went to my Headmaster who phoned around on my behalf and asked a neighbouring school, Thornhill High School, to register me. I finally registered Mathematics, Biology and Chemistry and had to forgo Further Mathematics due to the tricky financial situation and the limited time I had for study.

Two weeks later, I accidentally bumped into him again and he suddenly remembered that I had not paid my tuition and boarding fees. I conjured up an excuse and avoided him like the bubonic plague for the rest of the school term. I had considerable trepidation about bumping into Mr Nyanhongo. My heart would skip a beat whenever I saw him from afar in one of the corridors. My only consolation was that I came first in Mathematics, Chemistry and also as an overall class position at the end of the first term of 1997. Coming for second term was not necessary as the June examination started three weeks into the second term. I left a debt I could not pay at Fletcher High School and my 'dad's 30-year unfinished business' remained unfinished.

We could not afford to be in a hotel while I was sitting for my A-level examinations in Gweru, which were spread over a period of a month. My mom organised for me to sojourn for a month with her friend from the past. I sat my examinations while based at her place and went back to Bulawayo to stay with my uncle to await my results. After three months, the results came out and I travelled to Gweru to collect them. When I got to Thornhill High School and told them I was Hope, they said the Headmistress wanted to see me. And when she did, she gave me a good handshake, as she had not seen me before, and proceeded to give me my results. I had obtained the highest results and boosted the results from her school for the June examinations. I had got an A in Biology and B's in Chemistry and Mathematics. Biology had been my weakest subject and so I had given it more time at the expense of the other two. I was disappointed with the mathematics grade for someone who was doing A-level Further Mathematics.

University now beckoned and my 'dad's 30-year unfinished business' was at last done and dusted. To this day, none of my relatives or children from my neighbourhood in Mzilikazi in Bulawayo have ever surpassed by achievement in either O-level or A-level results despite my examinations being written in very trying times.

Chapter 5

Considering University

I N THOSE DAYS, fantasising about becoming a graduate professional required an inordinate amount of lateral thinking and thinking outside the box. Anything other than menial work was a pink elephant. The world we lived in did not have examples. My dad had been an accounts senior officer in one of the district offices and my uncle had become an electrician after undergoing years of apprenticeship at one of the largest biscuit-making companies in the country, the Lobels factory. My aunt had become a cook at a large referral hospital after completing an apprenticeship training following her Form 2 education (the equivalent of Grade 9 education) and my grandmum had been a Red Cross nurse assistant for decades. The trend in the neighbourhood was similar.

I cannot think of anyone of the generation of my parents, in the immediate neighbourhood of about two hundred houses or so, who completed a professional college diploma and had embarked on a professional career, with the exception of Magistrate Mapani. Magistrate Mapani was an established senior Provincial Magistrate in the city courts, and some of his court cases and judgements appeared in the national newspapers. He was employed in the mid and late 1970's as a legal assistant on a meagre salary at Lazarus & Sarrif Attorneys and learnt law in-house. He could not progress any higher because of the then colonial laws.

His fortunes changed dramatically at the Independence of Zimbabwe in 1980. There was a mass exodus of White magistrates soon after 1980 that almost crippled the judicial system in Zimbabwe. The University of Zimbabwe then moved to open its doors to any Black person who had 'any sort of legal knowledge' to enrol for a Diploma or Degree in law. Mapani jumped at the opportunity and enrolled in 1981 for the Diploma in Law. He completed the diploma within one year but had to drop from the degree programme because he had to fend for his family. He intended one day to complete the modules of the University of Zimbabwe but never did. He later chose and finished a long-distance correspondence Law Degree with the University of South Africa (UNISA) before joining the Judicial College of Zimbabwe to train as a magistrate. He began practicing as a junior magistrate in the small city of Kwekwe in 1982 and later in Kadoma city. He was promoted to serve as a Regional Magistrate in 1987 in the courts of Bulawayo, and later rose to become a Provincial Magistrate. He retired in 1998 and began legal consultancy. He sadly passed away in 2006. The lack of graduate professionals was a legacy of the colonial era laws and policies and had to some extent gripped the post-colonial kids.

So what on earth was I going to study at university? My career plans had been evolving over the years, which is normal I presume. In early primary school I had wished to be a shop teller. The shop tellers at 'Machipisini shops' in Mzilikazi took less than a second to work out the change after someone ordered say two loaves of bread and a pint of milk with a dollar coin. They were the 'kings of arithmetic' and in those days nothing was computerised or had the bar codes that are so prevalent today. The Zimbabwean Government was once a firm believer of price controls that made products very affordable and the shops were always packed with customers. Larger profits were made by the shop owners employing shop tellers who could shift the customers as quickly as a conveyer belt in a mass-production factory would do, for the profit margins amounted to only one or two cents per product. That is where the 'kings of arithmetic' came in handy. I loved mathematics!

My career fantasies in my later years at primary school oscillated in harmony with what the respective class teacher esteemed worthy goals, such as 'being a pilot' which surfaced in one of my 'when I grow up' essays. For some unknown reason, none of the teachers ever mentioned university. I saw myself as a technician in one of the factories repairing some equipment in my early secondary schooldays. Later on, from Form 3 onwards, my target was to get hold of a university science degree. The direction that was topping my career list during my A-levels was Pharmacy, or 'Pamacy', as I liked to call it. 'Pamacy' was a clean job working in air-conditioned places – air conditioned, otherwise the pills and drugs would deteriorate. Even the Zimbabwean Government financed vehicle loans to tantalise more people to take up 'Pamacy'. It was not too bad. All it took was a straightforward six semesters of fifteen weeks each to earn a Bachelor of Science Honours in Pharmacy, and so according to my very humble calculations, I would start the new millennium of 2000 as a Pharmacist. I got myself organised by booking appointments and meeting at least five different pharmacists. Fresh graduates of pharmacy tended to give most relevant and up-to-date university and employment information, and so those are the ones I chased up.

After I failed to sit for my examinations, in 1996, I decided to change my career path for the umpteenth time. I found routine work so nerve wrecking that I would have bravely climbed the thorniest tree south of the Equator than do routine work. Some people rather cherish the same routine work and would be perfectly happy stapling the lace holes of left shoes on the same desk of the same company for decades. The dread of Hope being stuck in some downtown Pharmacy for years bean counting 'panadol' or aspirin pills into prescription packets, over and over again and again, hit me like a ton of bricks. It was not to my liking indeed! I would not escape the bean counting of pills whatever workplace I might have chosen for my practice as a pharmacist. How hard would it be to count twenty-four pills into a packet, and could this not have been done by a primary school kid?

"Aaah nay" – and so I changed my mind.

I shifted my career goalpost to becoming a veterinarian from the months leading up to my re-sitting my A-level examinations up to the point of receiving my results. The range of animals from pets to big game requiring medical attention would have maintained my mental enthusiasm for a long time. Working in a private practice and occasionally taking the Landrover to care for some collapsed cow out there on the farms would have refreshed me. A newly built and swanky Veterinary Faculty, funded by the European Union, was up and running to ensure the country had sufficient technical capacity to supply beef to Europe and to be able to care adequately for the wild life in the national parks. Botswana had swallowed up a sizable chunk of Zimbabwean veterinarians and beef was its second largest earner from exports, after diamonds. However, I visited a couple of veterinarians and what they said was not encouraging. Apart from the fortunate few who got professional posts in veterinary medicine, a significant number of the most recent veterinary graduates had opted to teach in secondary schools out of desperation while the remainder spent their unemployment blues at home.

The honest truth was that Zimbabweans had no love for pets and they made no pretense about this fact. The dogs found in most large yards of Zimbabwean households were little more than efficient early warning systems to deter night-time burglars. No dogs were pampered by being allowed to sleep inside the house either. Brown stray dogs with slender elongated skulls roamed the streets and they had an acute sense of fear that made them break into a sprint at the earliest indication of someone posturing to pick up a stone to hurl in their direction. Limping livestock in the rural areas made their way straight into the cooking pot after anthrax or foot and mouth disease were ruled out. The only dogs in the country that drew some concern from the community were the missing dogs in the Warren Park suburb of Harare. Warren Park was a street opposite the site that was earmarked for the 40,000-seater National Sport Stadium, which was being constructed for the 1995 All Africa Games. The stadium was built by the Chinese and they lived onsite in a temporary camp. The camp became a one-way-traffic route for some dogs that "made fine cuisine", so we were told. There was no pet insurance available in the country. Thus, I sensed a limited scope for veterinary services in the country. That is how my love for a career in veterinary services came to an end. Nevertheless, there was a new kid on the block.

Physiotherapy was a new concept for the general public of Zimbabweans in the late 1990's. I read up what physiotherapy was at the local library, as it was before the internet age. I understood physiotherapy to be a branch of medicine that helped handicapped and disabled persons. All Physiotherapists in Zimbabwe were trained outside the country prior to 1987. The country then invested whole-heartedly and commenced a Physiotherapy degree programme at the University of Zimbabwe in 1987. A number of people helped in the early running of the physiotherapy programme and included Mrs Dorcas Madzivire and Mrs Jennifer Jelsma. Mrs Madzivire was the Vice President of the World Federation of Physiotherapists for a four-year term, in recognition of her contribution to physiotherapy in Zimbabwe and Africa. The programme required multiple sets of various electronic equipment, such as ultrasound and infra-red machines, tonnes of exercise equipment and consumables. It was mandatory that all the electronic equipment be regularly serviced. The Physiotherapy degree programme had an average of eighteen students per year. The new infrastructure and the small class sizes made the physiotherapy degree one of the most expensive degree programmes run by the University of Zimbabwe.

I first learnt what Physiotherapy is about in 1995 after having been informed about the degree programme by Kelvin Matingo, whilst still studying at Fletcher High. Kelvin, who was studying medicine at the University of Zimbabwe, lived about ten houses away from my house in Mzilikazi and had been a high school classmate of brother, Bryan. He excitedly nudged me about the acute shortage of physiotherapists in the country with the guarantee of employment after graduation. The first four generations of physiotherapists left the country to work in the United States of America. The employment agencies even had the nerve to offer employment contracts to second year university students in Zimbabwe. The agencies paid for the newly qualified Physiotherapy graduates to go and sit for the professional examinations in order to register as Physiotherapists in the United States of America. These activities soon caught attention of both governments of Zimbabwe and United States of America, who put pressure on the employment agencies to stop the further brain drain of Physiotherapists around 1998.

A new front was hatched in 1998 and Physiotherapy graduates found opportunities in the United Kingdom. The graduates had to sit for an examination to register with the Health Profession Council of the United Kingdom, but after a recognition of the standard and quality of the graduates from the University of Zimbabwe, this was waivered. The United Kingdom ran three-year Physiotherapy degrees that were less draining to the universities than the four-year Zimbabwean degree. The Zimbabwean physiotherapy degree programme offered additional clinical attachments and had a broader curriculum containing subjects such as joint manipulations. The clinical attachments of about twenty months of the four-year programme were spent on hands-on treatment sessions on patients, while students of the United Kingdom equivalent degree programme spent around eight months on clinical attachments. The United Kingdom degree programmes have the upper hand in being seamless and interwoven with the administrative and clinical departments of the National Health Service hospitals, and having well laid out tracks for progressive career development and the specialisation of Physiotherapists.

Before I wedded my life to physiotherapy by completing the university application form, I executed my homework. I paid visits to five physiotherapists in Bulawayo.[15] I rang up two separate Physiotherapists in Bulawayo; Ms Zoe Brest and Ms Madzorera, and organised ten minute appointments to get advice from them. Zoe's Physiotherapy Practice was at the eastern end of the central district of the city along Borrow Street, and the practice was very modern and tidy. Zoe employed three staff: a young secretary, a physiotherapy assistant (popularly known as 'Rehabilitation assistants' in Zimbabwe) and a messenger who doubled up as handy man for the practice. The secretary booked and maintained the records of patients and processed the paperwork to claim payments from the medical aid companies. Zoe was quite organized and she appeared on top of her game. I could sort of see myself in her shoes after half a decade or so later. It looked appealing.

Ms Madzorera's Physiotherapy Practice was in the southern end of the city, along 12th or 13th Avenue, and she had a significant load of physiotherapy home visits. The headquarters of the

---

[15]See map on page 6

National Social Security Authority, that rehabilitated workers who had sustained permanent injuries during work, was located in Mzilikazi where I had grown up, right next to Mpilo Hospital. I made an appointment to meet its head, Mr Sarashinge, a specialist Orthopaedic Physiotherapist who was either from India or Pakistan. I remember spending half a morning shadowing a physiotherapist called Julie at Mpilo Referral Hospital and another physiotherapist called Micheal at the United Bulawayo Hospitals. Virtually all the physiotherapists in government hospitals were in their twenties and looked quite cool and trendy. The job market did not look like it was going to be clogged anytime soon among the neighbouring countries either. Only Zimbabwe and South Africa trained physiotherapists among the sixteen southernmost countries in Africa. Almost the entire generations of physiotherapists of the 2003 to 2005 years are currently working in Namibia. It is rather heart-breaking to note that less than ten physiotherapists of the 500 odd graduate physiotherapists from Zimbabwe are still in the country.

The next logical step was to complete the university forms, which I duly completed in August 1997. My first choice was physiotherapy, followed by veterinary science, and pharmacy was my last priority.

Chapter 6

Gap Year before University

LITTLE DID I KNOW that going to university was going to be the least straightforward thing to do, especially after having passed my A-levels. I was about to unwillingly spend one and a half years before going to university.

After browning off for a few weeks until August 1997, I landed a temporary teaching post for four months at a school in the rural recesses of the Uzumba-Marambe-Pfungwe (quite a mouthful to pronounce!) District of Mashonaland East Province in Zimbabwe. It came just at the right time when I was saving up for university. I was to teach pre-O-level science and mathematics to pupils at Dindi Secondary School and that suited me well.

The school was a mission school run by the Methodist Church located in a very remote part of the district. The school was so remote that the bus came once a day and no wonder qualified science teachers had shunned it. The rural bus travelled from the school to the city once a day at five in the morning and another bus returned at around four o'clock in the afternoon. Free housing was provided by the school to all teachers. We had no water and electricity bills to pay because they were not necessary. A borehole and solar panels provided fresh water and electricity at the school. I ate goats like a hyena for they were surprisingly very cheap. I earned $2500 per month after tax and a full adult goat was a mere $80. Qualified teachers earned a net salary of $3500 but had less disposable income than myself because I did not have any dependants to look after. The downside was that the shopping centre was a decent 100km away in Murehwa town. We were given a day off to go every pay day to access our salaries in the nearest town, Murehwa. It took two months for a new government employee to be included in the national government payroll. I received my double salary after two months at the end of October in 1997. I used most of it to acquire things I would need for university.

There was a remarkable and critical incident that happened during my time at Dindi. I was in the throes of teaching Year 8 graders (Form 2 pupils) about global warming in a science class. The increase in carbon dioxide absorbs more of the heat from the sun which in turn melts a portion of the polar caps. The water from the melted polar caps would then submerge the coastal cities and people would need to move and live further inland. I stopped dead in my tracks when I realised that they all looked puzzled. The whole explanation was far too abstract for them and half the class did not have the faintest idea what iced polar caps were. I had never seen them either but had read about them. I drew a parallel of the polar caps to ice and the puzzled small faces dropped to a quarter of the class who vowed that they did not have the faintest idea what ice was! Most of the children had never been to the cities where they could have seen ice in a fridge or something. I dashed out to ask for an ice pack from the clinic, where it was kept for first aid and to store drugs at cool temperatures, and I placed an ice cube on each table. Some of the pupils were completely blown away by the slipperiness and coldness of the ice cubes. It was a whole experience for them and the way they stroked the slippery wet cubes made my day, and probably theirs too! It was only then that they understand the concept of 'global warming'. And so a teaching outcome that should have taken about ten minutes ended up taking a solid two hours. The country had O-level Cambridge examinations that had been set abroad by examiners who did not have a good grasp of the cultural day-to-day life of the examination candidates!

I was asked by the Headmaster to organise something for the end of the year Parents' day. I set up three activities run by students in one of the classrooms on that day. I set up an electrolysis station in which the bright blue copper sulphate solution copper-plated some simple nails. The other two activities were an IQ testing station and a demonstration of how soap is made from animal fat and caustic soda.

I returned to Bulawayo to sojourn with uncle Columbus after my teaching stint at Dindi Secondary School ended in December 1997 to prepare to attend the university which was opening for us in February 1998. I certainly miss Dindi Secondary School and perhaps one day I will pay it a visit.

After a few weeks I received a letter from the University of Zimbabwe. One of the greatest letters a youth can ever receive is a letter of an offer for a university place. My acceptance letter into a physiotherapy degree programme at the University of Zimbabwe duly arrived in January of 1998 and I was over the moon when it arrived. The administrators of the University of Zimbabwe then decided to move the opening date of the university to August and announced that they wanted "to be in sync with American and British universities". I was gutted and I had to find something else to occupy my time for the next eight months. My savings slowly eroded to nothing after a few months and I was feeling very fed up with the protracted delay.

It so happened that during one of my uncle's lunch breaks as he was chit-chatting on how happy he was with my examination results, his workmate expressed concern on how his two children were struggling with mathematics and uncle Columbus recommended them to me. They became my first private students that I taught and they lived outside my neighbourhood.

Word soon spread that I had passed my A-level sciences around the neighbourhood. One by one some parents approached me with the view of assisting and motivating their daughters and sons in pursuing O-level mathematics. There were now a handful of students in the neighbourhood who had achieved A-level grades to secure university places. Some of the pupils I assisted simply needed confidence boosting or perfecting approaches to examination, while some were pretty hopeless and were a good three years or more behind in their mathematical abilities. I bought a copy of their main mathematics textbook[16] to assist my tutorial planning. Not only did I love mathematics, mathematics returned my love. A loving smile would slowly spread across my face when my gaze into mathematical questions transcended into and grasped the 'beauty of mathematics'. I truly miss those romantic days!

A month later, I felt that I should fill my days with more students and placed a series of twelve worded adverts in the classified column of the local newspaper, the *Chronicle Newspaper*. The text of the adverts was *"O-level Mathematics tutor – in the comfort of your home. $Zim10/hour. Telephone 09XXXXX."* We did not have a telephone at home and mobile phones had just being introduced in 1997. Mobile phone charges were way too expensive at about US$1 per minute. I asked Magistrate Mapani for permission to use their telephone number for my customers to leave their messages. My students tended to be children born with a silver spoon in their mouths. Among the students I tutored were a daughter of a Black businessman in the Four Winds suburb and a son of an Indian businessman who owned a shoe shop in Lobengula Street. The son used to play a cricket video game on a computer in 1998 running Windows 98 operating

---

[16]*New General Mathematics for Zimbabwe* Book 1-4 by J.B. Channon, A. McLeish Smith, H.C. Head, M.F. Macrae. [Paperback] Publisher: Longman International Education ISBN-10: 0582079365 and ISBN-13: 978-0582079366

software! I had seen Nintendo video game hand consoles before but this was my first opportunity to see a video game running on a computer in someone's home.

On my first meeting with parents and student, I normally showed them my O-level and A-level certificates, together with my acceptance letter into the Physiotherapy degree from the University of Zimbabwe. I was proud of these three pieces of paper and they had become my gateway into the world of work. The certificates had become 'my magic passwords' in a way. I used to keep a small booklet as a journal track of lessons conducted. I made all my students sign at the end of the lesson, to avoid misunderstandings when writing a payment invoice at the end of the month. They usually paid on time. The money from the private lessons kept my wallet greased during the period of worsening inflation in Zimbabwe. Uncle Columbus never required me to chip in a little with the running costs of the home. He would be offended whenever I offered to help.

'I was a child,' was what he said.

The time to go to the University of Zimbabwe in Harare finally arrived around August of 1998. I sadly bade my students farewell and hoped for the best for them in the November O-level Cambridge examinations. I packed my belongings into two boarding school trunks and left Bulawayo a week before the orientation week. I sojourned at the home of my grand-uncle Musango in Mabelreign, Harare. Two nights after I arrived in Harare, much to my horror, I watched the news of the closure of the University of Zimbabwe. The handwriting had been on the wall for some months.

It would probably be a great omission to mention the closure of the University of Zimbabwe without mentioning a young man called Bornwell 'Warlord' Chakaredza. He spent about eight years studying for a three-year Bachelor in Social Science degree and never quite managed to graduate. He was obviously a smart guy and could have passed any examination had he applied himself. Instead he made his extra-curricular activities his main curricular activities. He was so heavily immersed in student politics and was the sitting President of the Students, perhaps for about three to four sequential years. 'Warlord' was suspended from the University a dozen times and each time he won the High Court appeal judgement allowing him back to University. By the time he came back, examinations were over and he had to repeat the year, and so that is why he took eight years to do a partial degree. He had a personal police riot helmet in his room on campus and rumour had it that he had initiated a duel with an armed riot policeman and conquered. He organised one of the most violent student protests that culminated in the riot police requesting the assistance of two military helicopters from the Zimbabwe National Army to bring the student protest under control.

The decline in economy over the last five years or so had slashed money in real terms available for higher education. 'Warlord' took full advantage of the feelings of neglect and disenfranchisement among the students. On numerous occasions, President Robert Mugabe bemoaned the behaviour of 'Warlord' on national television. However, the more Mugabe bemoaned him, the more it boosted 'Warlords' ego that he had caught the attention of the president.

I initially thought it was a simple delay of a week or so and so I stayed put in Harare, watching the evening news like a hawk! The Council of the University of Zimbabwe sat after a month and resolved to open the university in February 1999, some six months later. I was flabbergasted!

I felt it would be wise to start developing a steady portfolio of private mathematics students, to ensure a relatively steady income after I started university. I reassembled my advertising logistics I had fine-tuned whilst in Bulawayo. This time I designed a contract form and inserted a clause, which made the parents pay half the lesson fee if the child was absent on my arrival. I placed a series of adverts in the classified column of the Herald newspaper. My granduncle had a home telephone number which I used in the adverts. I was fully booked for about forty hours a week within a month. I taught mathematics to students in Form One to Form Four (O-level), to students at their homes. These homes were scattered throughout the length and breadth of Harare. I was so financially stable by October 1999 that I looked for accommodation. I was so mature for my age that I had the confidence to sign a lease agreement without a steady job. And so I entered an accommodation lease agreement, aged 19 years, with a landlord in Malborough (Harare) for 5 months before starting university and paid $US100 monthly. My sole financial income was from working as a part-time private Mathematics tutor.

I thank God I was offered accommodation on campus and the moving in date was February 1999. I gave my landlord the stipulated one month notice and off I went to the campus afterwards.

Chapter 7

Commencing at the University of Zimbabwe

T HE UNIVERSITY OF ZIMBABWE was the oldest, most prestigious and largest university in the land, the 'ivory tower of education' as it was known. There was nothing as magical as being at this university. Many, many years ago, Zimbabwe was part of the Federation of Rhodesia and Nyasaland. The then authorities had decided to build the first university to serve the three nations of Southern Rhodesia (Zimbabwe), Northern Rhodesia (Zambia) and Nyasaland (Malawi). Somehow, the lot fell on Zimbabwe and I am not sure why. With that being said, the university was opened amid much pomp and ceremony by her Majesty Queen Elizabeth in 1953. Princess Margaret had visited the country in 1952, the year that my mum was born, and was given her name.

I learnt later of the details of the opening ceremony of the University of Zimbabwe through a chat with Professor Phillip Tobias at the 17th Congress of the International Federation of Associations of Anatomists in Cape Town in late January 2009, which was their first Conference on African soil. Professor Phillip Tobias is one of the most eminent anatomists in Africa and has over 600 journal articles and 33 published books under his belt.[17]

A few days prior to the opening of University of Zimbabwe, the young Queen Elizabeth was in Bulawayo, my home town, to attend a 'Royal Orchestral Performance' there. "Oh, how Majestic she looked while seated on one reserved balcony," Professor Tobias recalled as he went down memory lane.

She then travelled on a three hundred mile long dusty road to Salisbury (later renamed Harare), the capital of Rhodesia (later renamed Zimbabwe) where the University of Rhodesia (also later renamed the University of Zimbabwe) was located. We were visually immune, as the locals, to the presence of the omniscient legendary dust of Zimbabwe. For newbies like the Queen, the dust cursed her crisply ironed white dresses into khaki shades that are reminiscent of ancient clothing found in museums. In a bid to ameliorate the dust, a convoy of water bowsers were to travel ahead of her entourage of vehicles and poured water on the road just before her vehicles came. It was in the shadows of the convoy of the Queen that Professor Tobias followed further behind and so became one of the least dusty trips to Salisbury.

My first day at the university was such a stressful day that it notched up my stress. The photo on my first year campus card bears testimony to the stresses of changing accommodation and moving into university residences, as well as the stress of starting a new degree course and the cultural shock of university life. Somehow, I soon learnt to adjust to my surroundings and activities.

The registration process was a real pain. The behemoth and inefficient registration procedure run by the administration staff

---

[17]http://en.wikipedia.org/wiki/Phillip_V._Tobias

of the University of Zimbabwe always reminded me of the Huang-He River in China. Huang-He perennially had floods on its banks and flooded houses, streets and farms, and the Chinese administrators never learnt how to get a grip on the floods, year after year. The whole process was like a long bottle with four bottlenecks embedded within the bottle. The registration form had tick boxes for the funding office, student accommodation office and new student campus card. Each tick box was in effect a queue bottleneck.

The first bottleneck was a queue to get the main student registration form from 'your friends'. The forms for each class were piled on numerous tables on the first morning of the five-day registration period. After the first morning there was complete chaos on this bottleneck. It was common for 'your friends' to find your form that had been trampled with a shoe stamp and shouting your name to draw your attention. You then continued searching for the form belonging to 'your friend'. About five percent of the forms were never printed and one had to travel four kilometres to the office of the Dean of the Faculty to prove that you were a bona fide student.

The next bottleneck occurred at the student loan funding office and was a genuine heartbreaker for many students. We had become the first students to pay part of the tuition fees up front. The students who could not raise the part tuition fees simply parked the registration forms in their drawers and attended classes as normal, while praying for a change of policy. Apparently about sixty percent of the students had failed to pay any fees and so it was not practical for a university to chase over half of its students halfway into a semester. Fortunately I had saved some money from my mathematics private lessons and paid the required $Zim3700, the equivalent of £300. Everyone who applied for the Government student loan was required as part of the application to provide certified copies of birth certificates and national identity certificates of both the applicant and parent or guardian. My cousin, Ian Musango, signed off my form as a guardian and surety for my student loan, as I had lost touch with both my parents for some years. I sent in my completed loan application and everyone waited for a decision for months on end.

Accommodation on campus was given to students depending on where they lived and could only accommodate a mere 20% of the students. The first years from outside the city had the highest priority and the last priority was for returning students from Harare. Nothing was guaranteed at the accommodation office and emotions ran high. The least dramatic bottleneck was queuing for the student campus card. If they took an unkind photograph of you, you were nevertheless stuck with a student card for the rest of the year that provided much needed comic relief to your classmates – if they ever saw it!

My memory goes back to the 'Baghdad' days. I was allocated to the New Complex 5, code named 'Baghdad' which was normally reserved for first years. Baghdad had an architecture of two circular building rings, each with three floors, that were joined by an open foyer. Baghdad had been the last student residence to be constructed and appears to have been built in a huff. There were some cracks here and there on the walls and the floors were evenly flat in some corridors. Baghdad had become the icon of student protests and demonstration against the overwhelming might of the Riot Police in Zimbabwe. The name Baghdad was chosen because Saddam Hussein had defied the odds and managed to resist the full strength of the United States of America army that was brought on by George Bush Senior in the 1990's. All the student protests were started by the senior students and they started their protests in Baghdad. Baghdad was near the north university perimeter fence and offered an escape route when the Riot Police invaded and descended on the campus.

In the breezes of February 1999 which brought a hint of rain, all the academic and non-academic departments started in full swing and were under pressure following the six months closure. There was no first year intake at the University of Zimbabwe in 1998, when I was supposed to start. As a consequence there were two first year intakes in 1999 and we had to do our first year courses in a record of six months, from February to July in 1999. We were given a token two weeks' rest between Semester 1 and Semester 2 of that year. The second batch of the first years of 1999 was sent acceptance letters to commence in August 1999.

Our Medical School was located in three geographical places. The preclinical departments of anatomy, physiology and biochemistry were housed on the main campus of the University of Zimbabwe, which was in the Mount Pleasant suburb of Harare. This was some six miles north of the Harare Central business area. The only available public transport to the main campus was in the form of some creaky privately owned twenty-seater buses which were normally stuffed with an additional ten standing passengers over and above the seated passengers during rush hours. The way we were packed in these full capacity buses never matched our dignity. We were jam-packed like sardines in a can!

The second part of the medical school housed the enchanted administrative office of the Dean of the Medical School, a fairly modern medical residence for the senior medical students and the clinical departments located in the northern end of Parirenyatwa Teaching Hospital. Parirenyatwa Hospital did not even try to conceal its physical size. It was the largest referral hospital in the country and had been named after the first Black medical doctor in Zimbabwe, Dr Tichafa Samuel Parirenyatwa (1927-62).

Tichafa had graduated in South Africa in 1957 and was appointed as the Medical Officer in charge of a mine hospital when he returned to Zimbabwe. He expectedly faced tensions from the nearby white mining and farming community whose familiarity with Black workers was only in doing menial and manual work. That mind-set hindered a healthy relationship and interaction between the farming community and Tichafa. He resigned within 4 years of graduating and entered politics fulltime as a Deputy President of one of the major pro-independence political parties. The loss of Tichafa was conspicuous and a gracious thank you letter from the local white farmers was tabulated in the local newspaper. Unfortunately, he died that same year in a suspicious car accident. When he died his body was brought to Mpilo Referral Hospital in Bulawayo. My grandmother from Mzilikazi, who apparently was a cousin of his, was called to identify him at the mortuary. She confirmed that it was him. What remains now is the fame of his name.

Racial status meant a lot. Each city in Rhodesia had two separate parallel health systems, one state of the art for Europeans and a basic one for Blacks. Parirenyatwa Hospital was formally known as Andrew Fleming Hospital and had been reserved for Europeans. It had much better infrastructure, while Harare Central Hospital had been for Blacks. As students we referred to the Harare Hospital as 'paGomo', which literally meant a hill, for the dusty hospital grounds and buildings sat on a hill. The 'paGomo' was the third piece of the Medical School puzzle and was right next to the high density residential areas of Mbare and Kambuzuma. Geographical units of the Medical School were harmoniously stringed together by a highly appreciated free 80-seater student bus that came around three times a day. The bus was nicknamed 'Zonke', the translation of the word from Ndebele meaning it was a very embracing bus and never excluded students.

All my first year courses were on the main campus (where I was living) with the exception of the Physiotherapy Techniques course, which required a ride on 'Zonke' to take me to Parirenyatwa Hospital. The Pre-clinical School of Medicine was on the southern end of the main campus. It was sandwiched between a ritzy new Faculty of Veterinary Science, which had been funded by the European Union, and the caged animals of the Faculty of Animal Science. The Faculty of Animal Science resembled a zoo of some kind, with baboons chattering away on that edge of campus. On the ground of the Pre-clinical School of Medicine lay the block with the Department of Physiology and Biochemistry on the right while the block with the Departments of Pharmacy and Anatomy lay on the left side. A huge newly built lecture hall, shaped like an aerodrome, lay near the entrance between the two blocks and at the furthest part lay a much smaller older lecture theatre.

Our class of physiotherapy and occupational therapy students was much smaller than that of the medical students and used a lecture room that was inside the block housing the anatomy department. We had an hour of lectures four days a week and the lecturers used a transparent projector to project their lecture notes onto a white rollable sheet that almost filled one wall. A carousel loaded with a circular magazine that held eighty 35 mm. square slides was used to illustrate the anatomical images. The slides had to be replaced upside down backwards and in the correct sequence, otherwise we would erupt into a giggle, when a wrong slide or an upside down slide popped up – much to the panic of the lecturer. We were taught by eight anatomy lecturers, mostly expatriates from India, Portugal, Bulgaria and Greece. Each lecture slot was followed by an hour of anatomical demonstrations on prosected specimens. The demonstrations were on human bodies that had been painstakingly dissected to highlight certain anatomical concepts and principles; especially the three dimensional nature of the human body. That was the order of the day.

Dissections were a very important teaching tool. Just imagine having a booklet showing six different photographic views of the foot; one from the top side of the foot, under side, inner side, outer side, front and a last one of the back heel of the foot. To reconstruct a three dimensional perspective might be a mental tangle for most students unless one held the actual foot with one's hand and rotated and saw all the views. It has been this very advantage that encouraged medical schools around the world to use dissected bodies, formally known as cadavers. Furthermore all the three hundred students studying anatomy were each given a full set of bones, as it is normal among medical students around the world, after paying a returnable token of deposit of $Zim70. Obviously many of the students carried human bones in their school bags and some bones on our study desks at home raised some eyebrows.

We had a notoriously grievous multiple choice marking on our anatomy tests after each anatomical region was completed and towards the end of semester. The marking scheme knocked off one mark for every wrong answer. In simple terms, if one got three wrong answers and seven correct out of ten questions, the three wrong answers cancelled out three correct answers leaving you with four out of ten (forty per cent) – a failure mark! The policy brutally rationed the distinction grades of brilliant students and only a couple ever got a distinction each decade.

Anatomy was perceived to be a difficult subject to get one's head around and had an overdose of exotic and unfamiliar words, and again perhaps twenty annotations on a single photograph or diagram. I had effortlessly learnt five languages over many years: Shona from home, Ndebele from my neighbours, English at primary school, Tswana during my holidays in Botswana and

French from High School. Now, I was being force fed the Latin-and Greek-laden vocabulary of anatomy at a breakneck rate of five thousand words over a period of six months. My response was spectacular and I would not recommend it for an average university student. I came to the conclusion that long notes taken during lectures, that duplicated the text book, was a luxury not worth spending time on. My Saturdays and Sundays were taken up with working as a private mathematics tutor and the money as a private tutor was my sustenance as a university student.

When I simply strolled into lectures the whole year with my hands in my pockets, without a pen or schoolbag, my classmates thought I was the biggest joke of the year and they could see the sinking of the Titanic. The strategy nevertheless seemed to work and I achieved top marks in anatomy tests that made up the continuous assessment. My main aim during each lecture was to understand at least four concepts very well from each lecture and not to have perfect notes that I would only make sense of when I got home. I had planned only to study my anatomy in three reading waves. The first wave was a familiarisation tour, the second was to prepare for the end of chapter test and the third was for the final examination at the end of year. My other first-year courses were Physiology, Physics, Sociology and Psychology. Physiology was about how the body functioned and entailed an understanding of hormones and molecular regulation. Psychology was about how the brain worked and Sociology illustrated how society was stratified and functioned.

The general atmosphere on campus among students was becoming restless and desperate. We had become the first generation to be paying market rates for food in the halls of residence that had just been privatised. Two months after starting university it became apparent that the government students' grants and loans were a mirage. The University of Zimbabwe had been one of the best national institutions that had propelled and fostered social mobility. The majority of students were from outside Harare, rural areas and smaller towns. The Bank of Mum-and-Dad was a simple non-starter for them.

The students from the more well off parents did not feel much of the financial distress that prevailed on the campus. I was not doing too badly either and had five regular students I was tutoring at their homes every weekend. Each lesson lasted two hours and the total time amounted to eighteen hours per weekend, including commuting time. I had no tutoring holidays throughout the year, lest my revenue nosedived. A student demonstration was organised by the Students Union leaders, led by Job Sakala and Learnmore Jongwe, who later became Members of Parliament. The demonstrations soon turned violent and damaged the campus supermarket, which was looted and ransacked, while the automated teller machine of Barclays Bank was vandalised. The action elicited the wrath of the Riot Police who descended onto the campus with teargas with a vengeance.

Chapter 8

Taking an Anatomical Career

ANATOMY WAS A WELL DEFINED DISCIPLINE and I could picture so clearly the arrangement of the structures. I seemed to excel in the anatomy examinations too. The great difficulty of mastering anatomy, and because it was a postgraduate qualification, ensured that there were less than five anatomists in the whole of Zimbabwe. It is always wise to enter a profession with a chronic shortage or inbuilt bottlenecks as it would guarantee jobs further down the line. I loved teaching too. I did enjoy the moments when I was a temporary secondary school teacher in the rural areas and a private mathematics home tutor in the cities of Bulawayo and Harare.

It was in high spirits that I started the intercalated Bachelor of Science Honours degree in Human Anatomy. The BSc Intercalated Honours in Human Anatomy degree interrupted and delayed by one year my four-year physiotherapy degree. Thus I spent two years studying physiotherapy, then took a gap year to study for the anatomy degree, graduated and then returned to finish the last two years of the physiotherapy degree and graduated again. The degree registration process was over in a blink, for it was for just the two of us. My colleague was a tall African lady from a private Girls High School in Bulawayo and was intercalating anatomy from being a medical student. We were given a large spacious office to share on the first floor of the anatomy building and had two executive desks and chairs, and had a blackboard to allow us to draw some of the most vexatious diagrams we bumped into.

We were extremely well looked after by Professor Levy, the Head of the Anatomy Department. We were given individual pigeon holes for receiving letters, free access to the staff anatomy library and could keep our food in the staff fridge. We hanged around and chilled out with the other staff members in the staff anatomy common room. We were also given a full cadaver to learn anatomy on and we each used one half of the body. The department made sure that we had individual microscopes, with the full complement of microscopic slides, which were allocated to us to aid our learning of histology. The anatomy technicians gave us unlimited access to learning aids and loaned us human bones. We were given a Pentium-1 computer with Windows 95 for use, which had previously been the computer of the anatomy secretary. The computers of the anatomy secretaries had since been upgraded to two Pentium-3 computers, which had the Windows 98 operating system installed.

The Pentium-1 computer was devilish. It had no USB port and only accepted three and half inch floppy drives of which each had a maximum capacity of 1.4 MB. The discs were exceptionally unstable and unreliable electronic storage devices that necessitated each research dissertation draft to be saved on at least four different floppy discs to spread the risk. In addition, the Windows 95 operating system was very unstable and laden with software bugs – once every hour or so the 'Blue Screen of Death' menacingly appeared, and the poor computer had to be restarted by cutting off its electricity supply and switching it back on. That meant the draft had to be saved every ten minutes or so when typing to prevent data loss and anguish of the soul. It was still far better than using a computer in the student area, which had more stiff competition for them and you had to stop typing at 4p.m. when they closed the computer laboratory.

The Government loan office only funded one degree and was not available for us to access, as we were embarking on a second degree. Professor Levy organised full scholarships from the John Trust, which was administered by the Vice Chancellor, Professor Graham Hill. The scholarship covered our stipend, stationary and some of the funds were earmarked for research consumables. Moreover, we were paid reasonably well for demonstrating anatomy to the medical, dental, physiotherapy and occupational therapy students. Shortly before starting the anatomy degree, virtually all my private mathematic lessons had dried up because of unrealistic hikes on commuter fares that had swallowed up my profit margins.

And so I sojourned with my granduncle in Mabelreign for a year during the anatomy intercalation year and moved out the following year. The study area at my granduncle's home was two metres in front of the television. My granduncle had a big heart, and eight adults and five children lived in the big house. I walked about three miles to the University each way for almost the whole year. The commuter 'kombis' offered a raw deal, for they only travelled half of the distance and with what they were charging, it was more sensible to put my feet into action and walk. I bought a 'Sony Walkman' to halve the distance and self-made cards with anatomy diagrams to keep me company. And they did!

Nevertheless, I had to put my best into my degree studies. The anatomy degree was divided into six components: advanced gross anatomy, advanced neuroanatomy, advanced embryology, advanced histology, comparable anatomy and a research project. Gross anatomy is the part of anatomy that can be seen with a naked eye and is the mainstay of cadaveric dissections. Neuroanatomy was about the parts of the brain and embryology was of how the unborn baby developed from a single cell. I found embryology most difficult and each and every sentence in the embryology textbook incessantly introduced a new word. I studied my histology by going through all the microscope slides with a history atlas once every two months. Comparative anatomy is the study of anatomy of different animals and was taught by a veterinarian anatomist, Doctor Mushonga. The biggest lesson I learnt in comparative anatomy was that human bodies are 95% similar to most animals.

Our learning objectives were carved out for us and it was to learn the anatomy of the body in and out. There were three different classes learning a different region of anatomy each week. We had to be very comfortable demonstrating in any of the anatomy practicals, irrespective of what the students were learning. We also had to write all the tests they wrote, so as to remove the fear of anatomy tests and demonstrating, at a rate of a test every two weeks.

I offered free demonstrations to second year medical students every Wednesday afternoon on whatever they wanted me to revise on. We had access to a cadaver and a blackboard available. These tutorials laid very solid foundations for my anatomical knowledge and also helped me gain contacts of private anatomy students the following year.

The year was soon over and the examinations arrived. We had four written examinations and one massive oral examination called a 'viva voce'. I had four lecturers grilling and quizzing me on anything in anatomy, and lasted an entire seventy minutes. A football match lasts for ninety minutes! Professor Levy kicked off the oral examination by strangely asking me about the 'Galapagos Island', where Charles Darwin had some of his scientific observations. I told him that I did not have the faintest idea where it was. Perhaps he was probing the breadth of my general knowledge. He proceeded to ask some neuroanatomical questions which I had no problem answering. Doctor Mawera was next and asked me about some X-rays of children, gross anatomy like identifying a certain nerve of the arm called the 'musculocutaneous nerve'. Doctor Rao took pleasure in asking me to identify the tissue on microscope slides which were intentionally poorly focused. He raised the bar by not allowing me to fine focus them and I motored on well on three of the four stations. It was the longest oral examination I was to ever have in my whole life and my nerves were so worn out after the gruelling seventy minutes that I felt like going to sleep, although it was only 11a.m. when the examination ended.

The University of Zimbabwe had absolutely no confidentiality in releasing examination results. The results were callously posted all over the university notice boards for the whole world to see and for whoever was willing to see them. If your friends saw your results before you saw them, they gladly told you that you had passed. If on the other hand if you failed, they left you to find it out yourself that you had failed some courses, or worse still that you had crashed out of university. On this particular occasion, they told me that I had passed. On arrival at the notice board in Pre-clinical Medical School, I found I had been awarded not only a 2.1 degree class, despite the grievous negative marking system, but also scooped the University Book Prize for being the Best Anatomy student. The graduation in the Bachelor of Science Honours in Human Anatomy degree followed a few weeks after the results were released, and on the next Monday I was back in class for the third year of the Bachelor of Science Honours in Physiotherapy degree. What an anti-climax it was!

At some point the following year, I was honourably called to attend the Faculty of Medicine prize-giving ceremony to be awarded the University Book Prize from the Vice Chancellor, Professor Graham Hill. Although the prize was a book token, it was an important landmark. It was a significant day for physiotherapists in Zimbabwe, for I had become the first physiotherapist to have been formally trained in anatomy. It gave confidence to the Anatomy Department to continue to take students from the physiotherapy and occupational therapy undergraduates. Furthermore it inspired a number of therapy students to consider seriously a career in anatomy as well. Since 2001 when I graduated, there has been a perpetual one or two undergraduates from Physiotherapy and Occupational therapy specialising in anatomy every year. My camera misfired that day. The film reel in my camera had sat poorly in the camera, which resulted in absolutely no photographic trace of the ceremony. However, this never quenched the excitement I had for that ceremony.

Chapter 9

Clinical Training as a Physiotherapist

THE SECOND YEAR OF PHYSIOTHERAPY threw me into the world of chest physiotherapy in late 2000. It was a side of physiotherapy I never knew existed. I had thought physiotherapy was restricted to sports, exercises and rehabilitation. Physiotherapists have an important but unenviable mandate of maintaining the hygiene and clarity of the lung tubes and the trachea of patients. An accumulation of mucus in the lung airways literally suffocates you by blocking air from reaching the lungs and the mucous is a heavenly hotel for bacteria to grow in. The bacteria would turn the colourless mucous yellow with their toxins and finally into a nasty foul smelling green phlegm. The lack of air would kill you in minutes while the build-up of bacteria toxins could be fatal a few days on.

The trademark instruments that all doctors have hanging around their necks is an instrument called a stethoscope and is used to listen to lung sounds. Listening to the chest with a stethoscope helps in locating where most of the phlegm is hiding in the lungs. Stethoscopes were compulsory for us and I bought a second-hand Littman type which I extended by an additional two feet using a nasogastric tube, a feeding tube inserted through the nose, that I freely picked up from the wards. The unlenghtened stethoscopes were giving me a backache. I had been of average height until the age of 17 years at Fletcher High School, when I shot up to a six foot four bloke like a weed within the space of three or four years.

All major surgery, pneumonia and any inability to clear the phlegm are a bad omen in that it means there is increased phlegm in the lungs. We used gravity and tilted the patient to drain the phlegm from its hideouts, and banged on the chest to speed things up. We were trained in special techniques to stimulate a coughing reflex from a patient. In cases where the patient was unwilling or unable to cough due to pain or heavy sedation, a special portable vacuum machine called a suction machine was used as the last resort. The sucking tube was placed either in the mouth or nose route and pushed further down until it reached the phlegm hideouts in the trachea. The mouth route was far more comfortable for the patient than the nose – just imagine the feeling of an insect buzzing and crawling up your nose! Chest physiotherapy is so important that hospitals usually have a physiotherapist on call on all evenings, weekends and bank holidays.

One patient I will never forget was a cute two-year-old girl with 'PCP pneumonia', a pneumonia typically found in immune compromised patients. During the first days tilting the body worked and the baby would cough out the phlegm. She grew drowsier with time, perhaps due to the prescription drugs or the heavier dose, and was slowly losing her alertness because of the fever. The parents had to call me one midnight from home and the dad picked me up, after fearing that the baby would not make it to the morning. When I arrived phlegm was making breathing hard labour and air was failing to pass the phlegm roadblock. I had to increase the frequency of my treatment sessions to five times a day including a ten o'clock session at night. At this stage, the special coughing technique was no longer working and I had to use a suction machine to clear her chest. I continued for a couple of days with her. On a Sunday morning I went to give her a lung cleaning before I went to church and I had told her mum that I would return after church. On my way back to the Children's Hospital, the dad telephoned me to say the child has passed away. I sat down, taken aback and wondered, 'What is the meaning of life?' It was rather disturbing dealing with the death of a patient to whom you had devoted so much time and effort and compassion and everything – a patient who in the end did not pull through.

My fourth of the five years in 2002 at the University of Zimbabwe was pleasant, and that was my third of the four years of physiotherapy training. The focus was on orthopaedics, the study of diseases and conditions of bones and muscles. Studying anatomy to a greater depth was an advantage for my learning of orthopaedics. The effects of different nerve paralyses or the directions that fractured bone fragments went were so much clearer with my greater acumen in anatomy. It was satisfying to be a reference person for anatomy related questions in lectures during my orthopaedic year. Whenever a lecturer or a presenter was not sure of some anatomical tangle, all eyes zoomed on me. We were graced with ten different orthopaedic courses such as sports injuries, restoring fractures, making plasters, treating nerve injuries, bone conditions of children and bone surgery. I had ample opportunities to watch different types of surgeries on patients. The Physiotherapy Department deployed us across the country for about four months of clinical attachments every year. I remember quite vividly observing several delicate surgical procedures, such as a repair of a hole in the heart, binding together a fractured thigh bone and a 'slipped disc' of the back. I am forever grateful for having had a training that was on patients, who appreciated the assistance they received from us and never entertained even half a thought to sue us.

The economic problems were getting worse in the country. The joy of being able to breathe in the country was becoming grievous and burdensome. Inflation shot up to 80% that year of 2001 and was compounded by a paralysed agricultural sector that was having serious teething problems after the land redistribution by the government. The manufacturing sector behaved with impunity and they preferred to increase prices instead of increasing production. The currency fundamentals grew weaker and in turn pushed up the prices of imported petrol almost weekly. The public transport was almost exclusively in private hands, and the owners were indifferent to the plight of commuters. The transporters had super knee-jerk reflexes and always hiked their fares higher than petrol price increases, despite petrol being only 15% of the operating costs. Inflation eroded the Government budget in real terms and social security nets sadly soon became excess to core functions of Government. There was no international assistance or redemption on the cards. The country became a 'persona non grata' for international financial institutions like IMF and World Bank.

We were a particularly vulnerable lot as students. We were not yet economically active, especially with some of our courses that took half a decade to complete. Early parole was for the inglorious university dropout and not a tentative option. We received government loans that were being pulverised in real terms after adjustments for inflation. The university administrators turned their backs on us and left us high and dry because they too did not have the financial muscle to subsidise the prices down. The university administrators privatised the dining halls, and dumped us at the mercy of the ruthless tycoons that were chasing after fortunes by overcharging student meals. I recall once that one of my classmates commented on the ridiculous prices for the finest cuts of prepared beef dishes. The canteens bled us white. The vast majority of students resorted to cooking in their rooms that had been purpose built for just studying. What else could they have done? The financial distress also affected the Physiotherapy Department, which in turn stopped paying our transport fares for going to other parts of the country. They resorted to limiting clinical attachment to within Harare only.

I survived largely unscathed by the national economic upheaval. I had my blessings. All it took to secure a temporary Junior Lectureship in Anatomy was a two-minute chat with the Head of Anatomy Department, Professor Levy, when I was about to start a three-month vacation. Professor Levy appointed me and I had a short stint between my third and fourth years of Physiotherapy training. On another vacation I was seconded as an Anatomy Demonstrator in Anatomy to the newly established medical school of the Bulawayo College of Medicine. It felt like a homecoming. I worked about half a mile from where I grew up in Bulawayo. The second three-month stint was prior to commencing my third year of Physiotherapy training. I left the Bulawayo College of Medicine a very disappointed man. I was told exceptionally long stories why they were not paying me, yet everyone else was getting their monthly salary paid on time. I was finally paid three months after I had left and not until my case had reached the desk of the Vice Chancellor of the Bulawayo medical school, Professor Chinyanga. The financial rosiness did not evaporate when I returned to attend my classes in Harare during the academic period either. I had a steady clientele portfolio of medical students requiring private tuition in anatomy on weekends.

The orientation for first year Physiotherapy students was almost non-existent for most of the years I was at the university. I joined hands with other students to organise an induction in 2000, while in other years, no one assisted and I proceeded solo. I briefed them on the main courses of physiotherapy, a bit on student finances, sources of cheap second-hand textbooks and a list of study skills they would need to acquire. I warned them to budget for some purchases. A white laboratory coat was essential for anatomy and physiology practicals, as was a stethoscope, for listening for chest sounds, and a name badge. Each student needed to have many sets of the blue and white physiotherapy uniforms during student attachments. The session ended by showing the students the cadavers they would be using for the year, and their anatomy and physiology lecture rooms.

My fifth year started with a unique opportunity to travel. I inadvertently came across an advert for a fully funded workshop in research techniques in brain research in Kenya. I was one of the two Zimbabweans chosen and got my first stamp on my passport just before boarding my first ever flight. It was hosted and funded by the 'International Brain Research Organisation' and at the time there was no postgraduate taught course in Neuroscience in Africa.

The last year of Physiotherapy was dedicated to brain conditions and disorders. The courses included brain surgery and physiotherapy of brain conditions. More than 50% of the year was spent on clinical attachments, including an elective attachment. I had opted to go to Botswana for a clinical elective for four weeks clinical attachment, but it fell through. I then went to St Anne's Hospital instead, one of the two major private hospitals in Harare. One of the weeks was spent giving physiotherapy at the week-long National Cottco High Schools Rugby Competition held at Prince Edward High School, attended by over 80 schools. I had a great time there and the bulk of problems were muscle ailments. The kids were so full of blood and energy, and boys were boys. I still vividly remember a young lad who collapsed after a head knock. On being brought to our First Aid tent, he woke up after a few minutes and started having two streams of tears meandering down his chubby face.

"I want to go back and play," he retorted with palpable zeal. We could not take any chances and we refused him to go back to the pitch.

My student days ended with my second graduation ceremony, which was held in the Great Hall of the University. We were capped and conferred with the Bachelor of Science Honours degree in Physiotherapy by the Chancellor of University of Zimbabwe, President Robert Mugabe. He was the Chancellor for all the state universities, about ten in all. As he was capping me he said an honest 'well done'. This was the only graduation at the university in about half a decade where he personally capped the graduates. He normally just waved to the entire classes to mark their graduation. Security was extremely tight and cameras were banned, in case some "James Bond camera 'sprung into action and coughed out bullets'." Sadly, once again I could not have a 'Kodak moment' of my graduation.

Chapter 10

Graduate Employment in Zimbabwe

A ND THERE WERE JOBS GALORE once yours truly graduated. A mere 18 Physiotherapists graduated every year from the University of Zimbabwe and the total in the country was less than 100 physiotherapists for a country of 10 million people. On the other hand, the United Kingdom had about 7000 physiotherapists per 10 million people. I landed a Junior Physiotherapist post for my residency at the Harare Referral Hospital. We were rotated to a different specialty every four months. My first rotation was in treating general out-patients and in-patients with fractures of bones. A rotation in children's physiotherapy was followed by a rotation in treating patients with brain and spinal cord conditions.

Simultaneously, after a two-minute chat with Professor Levy, I also got a teaching post as a Junior Lecturer in Anatomy at the University of Zimbabwe. A great time teaching anatomy it was, and I fondly used to re-tell my students the words of my former anatomy lecturer, Dr Prasada Rao. At times when Dr Rao taught a piece of extremely convoluted detail that left some clueless, he would say, 'Some will understand it now, some later and some will never understand it.' And at times, I used an equally cynical saying by an English Anatomy Professor who liked saying, 'Ladies and gentlemen, forget this if you can.'

Being a physiotherapist and also an anatomist allowed me to have a deeper understanding of clinical conditions in the hospitals and appreciate the importance of anatomical structures in real life scenarios. I was frequently consulted by my colleagues on puzzling cases that had a high component of clinical anatomy and surface anatomy. It was a joy to dissect a shoulder joint for students in the morning, treat a shoulder problem in the afternoon and explain the shoulder symptoms to the students the following morning.

I loved the clinical Physiotherapy world and that love still remains. Some days were downright monotonous, while some were heart thumping and amazing. At times, we just saw it as a job and forgot that it was 100% reality for the unwell patients. There are two outstanding clinical cases that have become etched onto my mind. For a person to have a stroke is perhaps one of the most humbling conditions that one can have. Half your body becomes floppy, your leg or arm no longer feels under your control but feels like it has been glued onto you. Round the clock care for everyday grooming becomes a necessity in severe cases. I have seen a number of patients who spontaneously start crying because of the immense helplessness they find themselves in. Although this condition is caused by the bursting of an artery in the brain, the effects are felt in the legs and arms. I had the unenviable task of explaining to elderly grandmothers and grandfathers in a vernacular language that a part of their brain was dead. I showed them a radiological image of their brain with a big blob on one side of the brain. I went on to tell them that although they were not insane or crazy, the blob has shut down control of their legs further down. Nevertheless, a number of them thought it was witchcraft, while some frequently put the paralysed leg in warm water at home in an attempt to bring it back to life.

My most heart wrenching case was of a 19-year-old boy who lived with his dad and stepmum. For very predictable reasons, he did not get along with his stepmum and his relationship with her had been sour for some years. Well, he decided to get himself out of the misery and tried to commit suicide. He tossed himself in front of a haulage truck and survived. The price was quite high. On arrival at hospital, the orthopaedic surgeon had no choice but to make amputations on three limbs. He made a left above elbow amputation, a right below elbow amputation and a right above knee amputation. As the physiotherapist in charge, I had no access to fancy prosthetic gizmos or gadgets. Crutches for amputation were not an option because he had no useful hands. Even to scratch himself on his back, he had to shout for the nurses to help him. I did all that I physiotherapically could have done but was still convinced he was conjuring up yet another suicide attempt. I tossed and turned at home thinking what suicide method a one-limbed teenager could use. I could not think of any. He badly needed a clinical psychologist and a social worker to work his case. One morning after coming to work, I found out that he had been discharged without my knowledge and I never saw him again. Such memories stay with you for a lifetime.

I am a firm believer in the doctrine of touring your backyard or area you live in before you tour faraway lands. During my annual leave in June 2004, I set sail for Great Zimbabwe and Victoria Falls, two of the five UNESCO World Heritage sites in Zimbabwe. I had seen the other two sites during my childhood which are in the vicinity of Bulawayo – Matobo Hills and Khami Ruins National Monument. Great Zimbabwe was a 12th century city, the oldest and largest in the whole of Southern Africa and served as a royal palace for the ancient Zimbabwean monarch.[18] Great Zimbabwe was a city of 20,000 people and was built out of well calculated interlocking large stones, with each stone weighing about ten stone. Great Zimbabwe literally means

---

[18]http://en.wikipedia.org/wiki/Great_Zimbabwe

'house of stone' and gave rise to the name of the country at Independence. Where the builders got the stones from, who carried them, how they were carried are unanswered questions, and are part of the legacy of the ancient city complex. They believed in the spiritual world and hence were a city without an army. No one knows why it collapsed.

From Great Zimbabwe I trekked to Victoria Falls and passed through Bulawayo. I booked four days at a lodge in Victoria Falls. How memorable it was having a sunset cruise a hundred yards before the mighty falls of the Zambezi River, Africa's fourth longest river.

After finishing my year of physiotherapy internship, I was issued with an open Practicing Certificate by the Medical Rehabilitation Council of Zimbabwe. My aspiration would be to assemble enough capital to set up a chain of charitable Physiotherapy clinics within lower socio-economic urban communities. I would like to target specific conditions like cerebral palsy in children or strokes in adults. With this I envisage a time when it will be possible to link up with like-minded persons and organisations in order to set up the infrastructure, vision and desire for the best service possible. It is a blemish on our hearts as physiotherapists from Zimbabwe that although 80% of us come from the lower socioeconomic levels and trained our skills on poor people who come to Government hospitals, that once our skills have been perfected, we shun the lower socioeconomic groups. Most of us have gone into private practice to cater for the wealthy or have gone abroad to ply our trade. There are no easy answers either. For a little while longer, while we collectively hatch a credible plan, we hope our patients will be patient enough.

I enrolled for an English course that was a prerequisite for registering as a Physiotherapist with the United Kingdom Health Professions Council. A few months later, I registered as a Physiotherapist with them. We needed no physiotherapy examinations as Zimbabweans, because our country had a compatible education system to the United Kingdom educational system. The University of Zimbabwe was originally set up as an affiliate college of Oxford University, with the medical school being affiliated to the medical school of the University of Birmingham. The constitution of the University of Zimbabwe was literally a photocopy of the Oxford University constitution. All the pupils across the country sat O-level and A-level Cambridge examinations.

Towards my last days in Harare, I was invited for a week-long academic conference in Rabat in Morocco. After changing flights in Dubai, I headed for the Moroccan capital, Casablanca. The Arabic country felt so exotic, even the road signs were in Arabic. The country had been colonised by France and perhaps only people who had high school education spoke French fluently. I brushed up the French I learnt at Milton High School and it came in handy. I enjoyed Moroccan cuisine which was delicious enough, although we had to be careful because we were told they ate horses, which we abhorred. We were worlds apart in the linguistic department and we resorted to mimicking the noises of the animals just to double check there was 'no horsey business' on our plates. The hotel we were booked into lay a few metres from the coastline of the Atlantic Ocean. It was my first ever time to dip my hand into the Atlantic Ocean. Memories of walking through the 'medinas', fortified old cities, kindle fond times. There were some strange habits in Morocco. I could not work out if it was the love for their king or compulsive laws that made each and every public building shop or tuck-shop display the portrait of King Hussein. Morocco is one of the last true kingdoms in Africa so it has no president.

Chapter 11

Modernity and Legacies of London

MY FIRST EVER RENDEZVOUS WITH LONDON was in June of 2004. I was on my way to Norwich where I had been short listed for an Anatomy lectureship post at the University of East Anglia. Unfortunately there was a stronger candidate and I missed the job. I spent a single week in England and returned home to Harare feeling low spirited. One night was spent in Norwich and five nights in London with my aunt. Most of my friends were quite surprised I had come back so quickly after spending a fortune flying halfway across the planet. I had told them I was going for a week and sure enough I was back after a week, and I could not understand or decipher their surprise.

My second visit to England was in December of 2004 for research collaborations at Bristol University. I used my annual leave days from work. My biggest surprise was that there was no snow in London on Christmas day. Professor Levy, a neurosurgeon, had supervised my research which was to find out why people developed 'slipped discs' on their backs. 'Slipped discs' are an extremely painful and very disabling condition. They are caused by the oozing out of the contents of intervertebral discs located between each pair of back bones onto major nerves of the legs.

In the 1960's Professor Levy was confronted by a medical puzzle that continued to nibble at his mind for the next four decades. He had surgically repaired 'slipped discs' on a thousand White people but only came across 16 cases among Blacks over a ten-year period. Professor Levy suspected that the anatomy of the backs of Blacks and Whites was different, especially the muscles. Forty years later in the year 2000, Professor Levy asked me to collect a tally of all the 'slipped disc' operations in Zimbabwe of a five-year period from 1996 to 2000. In addition, I was to dissect and compare the anatomy of the backs of Whites and Blacks that were in our Anatomy Department of the University of Zimbabwe, to try and find clues to solve our case. Upon analysing the results, the anatomy of the backs of Whites and Blacks were like two peas in a pod. The number of surgical operations across the country were neck to neck in numbers for the two groups. So it made sense to inquire further and to seek new insight from the expert at Bristol University. I had research collaborations with one of the eminent researchers on the human back and I returned to work in Harare after the collaborations.

In early 2005 I landed a job in London. The company applied for and received my work permit from the Home Office of the United Kingdom to enable me to work for them. The company posted the work permit to me in Harare, which I used to apply for and obtain a working visa clearance from the British High Commissioner in Zimbabwe.

London seemed so full of life. London has people from 208 countries although the United Nations only has 168 countries. The insightful sense of modernity was surprisingly at ease with centuries of the legacies of the British Empire. The love of old buildings was part of the DNA of London. I expected buildings like Westminster and Buckingham Palace would still have the ancient architecture and bricks, but not on the newly built residential homes. The new London homes were usually adorned with 'dirty bricks'. The 'dirty bricks' were simply newly made bricks that were decorated or painted to make them look like they were hundreds of years old.

The seats on the London Underground trains certainly looked first class and I was easily swept away with the way the Londoners tapped their oyster cards. The machines deducted the correct fare in a split second before the gates opened to allow one to pass through. Nevertheless, working out the right train route was more like a gamble for me and it was initially difficult to go to the appropriate platform. I could not get the hang of the correct direction in terms of west vs. east-bound or north vs. south-bound trains when they arrived at the platform. With time, I got the hang of it.

Londoners were unusual in some regards. The silence of commuters in London Underground trains was so surreal. The unwritten rule is that you do not chat with anyone on the trains. Half the passengers stuffed white earphones of the newly released iconic iPod player into their ears. The rest either juggled their emotionless faces and cheeks in synchronisation to the rumblings of the train, read thick novels, or the free 'Metro' newspaper. Londoners were so detached from each other. Back home people usually chatted light-heartedly about recent social developments or about the weather in order to break the chat ice. For us chatting among ourselves while commuting imparts a stronger feeling of trust and belonging to the community.

And London, being very competitive, probably has the highest percentage of people with degrees, which is almost 50% of all adults. Londoners are a relatively younger lot who do not normally mind working overtime hours. I reckon that if a young lad can survive in London for a couple of years, then he can probably survive in any city.

It is a normal tradition for all newcomers to the United Kingdom to have "chicken and egg" problems when trying to open a bank account. If you have a chicken, they want you to wait until it lays an egg, and if you have an egg, then they would want you to incubate it until you have a chicken. The banks require proof of where you are living, like a water, electricity or land phone bill, to open a bank account. On the other hand you need a bank account for any company to pay you your first salary, for without it they will not pay you. I lived in accommodation provided by the employer and had no chance of having a water, electricity or land phone bill in my name. Even if I had not lived in the accommodation provided by the employer, a utility bill in my name would only come once I signed a lease agreement after paying a deposit. The deposit however is impossible to pay because my employer will not give me my salary because I do not have a bank account. Somehow, somehow I broke the vicious circle and ended up managing to open a 'no frills' Lloyds basic bank account. It only worked with Lloyds ATM machines and did not allow me to purchase anything at supermarkets. Lloyds Bank sent me my first bank statement after a month or so, and that was the document I used to open my first proper Barclays Bank account, that could allow me to buy things at the supermarket and online on the internet.

It was whilst I was in London that one of the largest terrorist bombings carried out by four home-grown British Islamic fundamentalists took place, the worst incident since the Irish Troubles in Northern Ireland (from 1968 to 1998). Three of the four bombs went off in three different underground trains in London in a space of fifty seconds during the peak of the morning rush hour. One of the trains was blown up while it was about a hundred feet deep underground. The fourth bomb blew up a double decker bus to shreds an hour later. All mobile phones lost their network signals within minutes of the blast due to either congestion of the network by people calling for help or the authorities wanting to disorientate the terrorists. We could not tell which of the two applied.

The bombing changed the character of the police service to be on permanent high alert, although on some occasion they over reacted and this resulted in the death of Jean Charles de Menezes.[19] He was shot seven times in cold blood at the Stockwell Underground Station in London after being mistaken for a terrorist by the police. The London Police paid compensation and apologised to the family.

I received numerous calls from within the United Kingdom and from Zimbabwe from people inquiring after my welfare, including the secretary of the Veterinary Department at the University of Zimbabwe, whom I least expected to hear from. Since then, I have felt uneasy whenever I use the London underground trains.

It was hard working in London and I felt work was getting very monotonous. I felt it was now time to switch from Physiotherapy to Anatomy as an academic. I always felt that on the African continent is where I would find people and institutions with the patience to develop and nurture early talent. So to Africa I set my mind. Courses for Master degrees for Southern African students in South Africa were about 10% of United Kingdom prices. I chose the university with the highest ranking in Africa, namely the University of Cape Town, and I soon got in contact with Professor Jelsma and Professor Louw. I had saved up enough money to take me through one year of the two-year Master of Anatomy degree. I literally had 'to endure' the student visa application to South Africa. It took about three or four visits to the South African embassy in London. Part of the process was paying a security deposit of a whopping £600 and being zapped by an x-ray machine on my chest, to rule out chest TB. After I got the visa stamp, I resigned from work and made void about

---

[19]http://en.wikipedia.org/wiki/Death_of_Jean_Charles_de_Menezes

three years on my United Kingdom work permit visa, which was still valid for about three years. I shipped my goods to Cape Town and bought a one-way ticket, which was about 90% of a return flight. I was convinced following my 'passion' was the right thing to do.

Map of Southern Africa

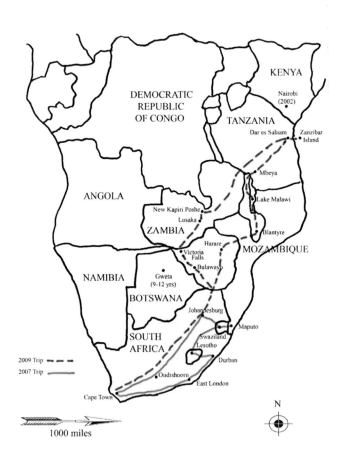

Chapter 12

Research Grooming in South Africa

I LEFT HEATHROW LONDON on a one-way flight ticket in March of 2006 for Cape Town. I had never been to South Africa before and it was a big step into the unknown. The University of Cape Town put me in touch with a taxi driver who normally collected international students. Sure enough, he was there at the airport with an A4 sized paper with 'Hope Gangata' written on it. I was quite excited and relieved to see him. I collected my luggage from the airport after customs clearing and packed them into his car. My heart sank when we were driving from the airport to the campus for the surroundings took me by total surprise. The airport was surrounded by an unsightly welcome for visitors – the shanty-towns of Gugulethu and Nyanga.

The free open spaces in the cities of South Africa, like the surroundings of the international airport of Cape Town, had attracted the rural folk to try their fortunes in major cities. The pitching of shanty accommodation in South Africa does not need any city planning approval at all. It is mostly because the local governments are avoiding a nasty collision course with the electorate and would like to please them. Apparently, the South Africa laws do not allow the police or any administration to remove people without giving them a humane alternative accommodation, which of course is expensive to give away. The complacency of the local government ensured a steady stream of newly erected shacks popping up every week. The public service arms of Government like water, sewage and electricity were always two steps behind. There was always a fresh quota of shacks they could not tear down yet had to connect to the national grid of water and electricity.

The setup of cities was different across the Limpopo River, the border that separated the countries of South Africa and Zimbabwe. Zimbabwe had no shacks with hundreds of thousands of people living in them. I had not seen anyone I had known living in one. Virtually all the houses across the country were of 'bricks and mortar'. Almost everyone in the world sadly remembers seeing on their newsreels 'bricks and mortar' houses being torn down by bulldozers in the 'Operation Drive Out Trash' in Zimbabwe in 2005. It was an attempt, without any warning at all, by city councils to deal with the rapid growth of urban populations. It was the norm and standard protocol for all the houses to have at least a full acre of ground around each and every house in Zimbabwe. Houses in less affluent and older residential areas almost exclusively had a tendency to build an extra bricks and mortar building on their yard without approval from the city council. The 'backyard extensions' generated some extra revenue for the landlords and eased the housing problem in the cities. Indeed, house rentals in Harare are one of the highest in Africa because the population growth has not been matched by new houses being built. The ratio of these 'backyard extensions' were as high as one to one with the official houses and were amply connected to the national water and electricity grids.

Out of the blue all the city councils across the country decided to liquidate the 'backyard extensions'. Teams of officials from the city councils with bulldozers, backed up by the police, were given the official maps of houses that had planning permission. They simply razed to the ground any 'new additions'. The residents of the houses came back from work only to find their houses looking like tombstones! A fact-finding report from the

United Nations mission noted that *"Unable to squat on public land, low-income urban dwellers resorted to what is commonly referred to as 'backyard extensions' of legal dwellings. These extensions, many of which were built with durable building materials and on serviced plots, proliferated as a form of affordable rental housing catering to effective demand by the majority of the urban population and providing a source of much needed income for their owners."*[20]

I now find it understandable why the South African Government is hesitant on tearing down any illegal shack. The pain would have been greater if the shacks had been made of more durable materials. My introduction to South Africa from the airport was such a great misrepresentation of the other brighter and glorious side of South Africa that lay beyond the shanty towns.

I soon arrived at the main campus nestled on the lower slopes of the famous Table Mountain, a site rated by UNESCO as a World Heritage Site. Table Mountain and its attendant peaks, Devils Peak and Lion's Head, are the most enduring images of Cape Town. The Table Mountain Park covers three quarters of the Cape Peninsula, trebling the demand for residential land and house rentals of the remaining quarter, and stretches from the flat topped Table Mountain to Cape Point some 15 miles away. One needs to see such sight. The two hundred year old University of Cape Town is probably the oldest in Africa and, indeed, has had ample time to achieve the distinction of being the highest ranking university in Africa. The University of Cape Town is ranked higher at number 103 than the University of East Anglia, which is at number 145 in *The Times'* top 200 universities in the world.[21] The University of Cape Town is now at the brink of

---

[20]http://ww2.unhabitat.org/documents/ZimbabweReport.pdf
[21]http://www.timeshighereducation.co.uk/world-university-rankings/2011-2012/top-400.html

entering the top 100 universities in the world. I soon arrived at the charming main campus of the University of Cape Town and it was a sight of sheer beauty. The backdrop of Table Mountain National Park blended with the beauty of the elegant buildings of the University of Cape Town.

The scenery from the University of Cape Town was stunning and the campus was well planned out. The main campus was arranged like five 'rice paddies' planted on the sides of a mountain. The first level had a flurry of about twenty tennis courts and was surrounded by tall waving pine trees. The academic and teaching buildings were on the next 'rice paddy', which was about two hundred yards or so away. There was another lower 'rice paddy' with the library a further fifty yards away, which had the great hall, food outlets and it also contained the main street of the campus. After that came the 'rice paddy' with two rugby fields on an even lower level. Upon the last and lowest 'rice paddy', a further two hundred yards beyond, sat the pretty main administrative buildings, the offices of the Vice Chancellor and the Law Faculty. There was a rather efficient free shuttle bus system available for students that threaded together the main campus, the Medical School, Law Faculty and the 'Hiddingh campus' of Fine Arts.

The century-old Medical School was on a different foothill of the same Table Mountain. The Medical School gained fame and praise by winning the race to conduct the first open heart surgery in 1967, with a team led by Professor Christiaan Barnard.[22] There was another notable discovery, at around the same time, of the invention of X-ray computed tomography, usually referred to as CT scans. CT scans are now used by almost every hospital in the world to see injuries inside the human body. One of the two inventors was the South African-born physicist Allan Cormack

---

[22]http://en.wikipedia.org/wiki/Christiaan_Barnard

who was later awarded the Nobel Peace Prize for his profound contribution to medicine and science.[23] The same laboratory is currently developing the latest breed of X-rays that reduce by 95% the amount of radiation given to a patient using a machine called a Lodox/Statscan®,[24] when compared to a normal X-ray machine. The new Lodox/Statscan® can scan the whole body in 13 seconds and has been adopted across the world as the best imaging to use to identify multiple injuries in Casualty Departments of hospitals.

I cherished each and every morning when I entered the Anatomy building and could not get enough of glancing over to see the Table Mountain National Park, dotted with an abundance of wild life, like the zebras, springboks and wildebeest. There was an ongoing ambitious project, running independently of the university, of resurrecting the extinct antelope, the quagga, on the national park. The quagga had become extinct from our planet for over a century. One of the last quagga to be shot dead had its hide kept at the Cape Town Museum. Some 'smart Alec', Reinhold Rau, in the 1990's decided to have a look at the hide and sure enough he found a tiny morsel of the dried flesh still attached to the hide. He ran a full DNA analysis and bang! What did he find? The DNA was exactly like that of a zebra. The only difference was that the quagga had faded black stripes on the back half of the antelope that finally became plain brown like that of a donkey. A photograph of a quagga was taken in a London zoo in 1870 and can be seen on the Wikipedia website.[25] So they looked for a pair of zebra with the brownest back halves and began selective inbreeding of them. I am excited because I think they have rekindled the lost quagga. Compelling pictures of

---

[23]http://en.wikipedia.org/wiki/Allan_McLeod_Cormack
[24]http://www.lodox.com/index.html
[25]http://en.wikipedia.org/wiki/Quagga

the newly bred 'quagga' can be viewed on the internet.[26] The whole project had a Jurassic feel to it and appears to have brought back an extinct animal.

The students learning anatomy dissected within the Anatomy Building. The students without fail cleaned their instruments after they had finished their day's work. They would wrap up the cadavers with care, dispose of their gloves and wash their hands. Massive two-foot wide tissue paper rolls were used by the students to dry their hands. The hall was at its noisiest period when filled with a hundred excited medical students. Some discussed how to proceed with the dissections while others were busy interpreting or misinterpreting the dissection manual. It was common for some to talk about the television drama of the previous night while others gossiped like extended families about their new boyfriend. The noisy air vents that sucked air with vaporised preserving chemicals, notably formalin solution, cranked up the decibels.

The physiotherapy and occupational therapy students had their lectures in a different building, while their dissection hall was in a smaller anatomy laboratory in level two of the Anatomy Building. It is worth noting that the students in the therapy class were far more relaxed and easy going than the medical students in dissecting practicals. The chilled-out attitude had rubbed off from their anatomy lecturer, Dr Christopher Warton. He was the most laid back lecturer I have seen.

Dr Warton is one of the few well rounded people I really admire. There are three 'time jewels' that are very dicey to juggle together for most people. A full-time job will chew at least thirty-five hours weekly. The time invested in being a member of a church fellowship (which involves attending prayer meetings,

---

[26]http://media1.mweb.co.za/quaggaproject/family3a.htm

church services, bible study), and the attendance of sport or meetings of hobbies, will surely swallow up another ten hours or so. Having a wife or a husband and young children in the home will surely mop up whatever time might remain of the week. People without all three commitments have it a bit easier, time-wise, as they just have to juggle family or work. It is not uncommon to hear of workaholics who have postponed having a family in order to concentrate on grooming their career.

I have only seen a couple of people who have balanced these three sparkling jewels so well. Indeed very few people have surpassed the example laid out by Dr Warton. He is married to his lovely wife of thirty-four years, with whom he has six children, of whom three have passed through university and all have studied theology. They are planning to celebrate their 35th wedding anniversary next year. Being practicing medical doctor accounts for a good part of his day time. Chris is involved in research into the changes in brain anatomy in foetal alcohol syndrome and has been graciously teaching anatomy for the past thirty years or so at the University of Cape Town. He painstakingly wrote a complete set of eight anatomy textbooks that he uses to teach physiotherapy and occupational therapy students. His anatomy teaching has been so thorough that he was awarded the 'Distinguished Teachers' Award' by the university for outstanding teaching standards. He still has time to inspire students while teaching medical ethics at the Bible Institute of South Africa Theology School. On any day he seems to have a smile and enjoys every moment of his life juggling his family, work and community church involvement.

Dr Warton, who is sixty and close to retiring, had to sacrifice achieving numerous journal publications and working towards being a professor or head of department, so as to maintain the balance. His wife is a qualified lawyer but sacrificed her career to be a full-time mum for her six children. A recipe for disaster is having things all over the show pulling in all sorts of directions. Imagine a young man who is studying in Norwich, has a girlfriend in Glasgow, a child in London, a part-time job in Cambridge and is actively involved in a church in Great Yarmouth. He is simply pushing his luck too far even with the best of intentions to level the balance. It takes prioritising what is important and has the most impact on your life so that you will not falter. Taking on things one at a time after evaluating to see if you have enough capacity to take them on is a handy hint. At a later time there might be a better chance that major things in your life become synergistic rather than a clashing impediment to your daily life. No wonder I have delayed finding a wife. I cannot wait to visit Dr Warton's family in Cape Town!

My keenness to prepare myself for mentoring university students and to get an abridged perspective on student life led me to take up subwardenship. I became a subwarden at the senior residence of Liesbeeck Gardens of the University of Cape Town, which accommodates about 500 students. The subwarden played a semi-parental and advisory role for the students who were living far away from their home city or home country. I would be woken up dead in the middle of the night to deal with residents who had lost keys and people needing to go urgently to hospital. I calmed rowdy folks when called upon. I was a no nonsense subwarden and I squirreled away the highest tally of noisy radio speakers after issuing firm warnings, probably about six. Subwardens had to be formally informed if a resident was going to have an overnight visitor, otherwise a tip off would trigger surprise 2a.m. squatter raids. The unwelcome 'visitor' was unceremoniously accompanied to the outside perimeter of the residence by the university security personnel during the middle of the night.

The demographics of the residence were quite remarkable. South Africa had just emerged from the jaws of an inhumane racial political system which had permeated every strand of civic society. The residential areas were still racially demarcated and so were the schools in them. Universities, such as where I was the subwarden, became one of the institutions where the average South African youth lived and learnt with other fellow South Africans of a different race. It was a steep cultural learning curve for everyone including yours truly!

There was always a good representation of international students from other worldwide places such as South America, Asia, Africa and Europe. The Liesbeeck residence received forty or so American students on an exchange semester. The largest group of international students was surprisingly from Zimbabwe and were actually 20% of all international students (IAPO May 2008 report[27]). The diversity of the city itself was remarkable too; about half of its four million population are of mixed race, who are more inclined towards Islam and surprisingly the Black Africans are a minority in this African city. Cape Town inherited a more vibrant and varied cultural theme than any city elsewhere in the world.[28] My experience as subwarden in such a city was a very valuable hands-on social experience.

Cape Town is the most popular tourism destination city in Africa and for good reason. The sheer size of the city tourism industry, with a comfy 60,000 bed capacity, increases the cultural vibe by temporarily having people from all over the world. The season, with its annoying rain drizzling in winter followed by scorching summers, is quite the opposite of my childhood climate of dry winters and wet summers. A 350-year-old lighthouse at Cape Point marks the blending of the warm Agulhas current of the Indian ocean with the cold Benguela current of the Atlantic ocean. My name's sake, the windy and rugged Cape of Good

---

[27]http://www.uct.ac.za/downloads/uct.ac.za/apply/intstud/apply/IAPOnews06-08.pdf
[28]http://en.wikipedia.org/wiki/Cape_Town

Hope, lies a mere mile from Cape Point.[29] The Kirstenbosch
Botanical Gardens present and celebrate the unique national
vegetation of the region as one of 'the most stunning gardens in
the world'. Robben Island, where the apartheid Government had
imprisoned Mandela, is just seven miles off the coast of Cape
Town. World class museums such as the District Six, Slave lodge
and Jewish museums grace the city. The wine farms and safari
parks are less than an hour's drive from the city. Quality beaches,
one foot tall African penguins in Simon's Town, the Waterfront
and the dock adorn the coast, while the ocean offers deep sea
fishing, dolphins, whales and sharks. You will never get bored in
Cape Town.

The origins of Cape Town can be traced back to the setting up of
a medical base to combat scurvy among sailors travelling from
Europe to India in 1486.[30] Mortality was horrendous and about
70% of the sailors died on the two to three months journey to
reach the Cape from Europe.[31] The treatment for scurvy was
simply fresh fruit. The settlers, who initially settled on the coast,
later moved inland primarily for agricultural land and many
tenacious battles were fought with the various inland tribes, like
the Zulus, Xhosas and the Hottentots. Diamonds, gold and other
minerals were later found inland and further inflamed the
tensions. Cecil John Rhodes and Alfred Beit rose as the leading
mineral tycoons from the heap of mining chancers. Rhodes later
became the Prime Minister of the Cape Government. Zimbabwe
was initially named after him, and was called Rhodesia for
several decades. Six statues of him were mounted in the different
cities where he had influence upon his passing away. Two statues
were mounted in Cape Town. There is a statue of him sitting at
the bottom of the Jammie stairs, which is on the part of the land

---

[29]http://www.sanparks.org/parks/table_mountain/tourism/attractions.php
[30]http://en.wikipedia.org/wiki/Cape_Town
[31]http://en.wikipedia.org/wiki/Scurvy#18th_century

he donated to the University of Cape Town, and another of him standing located at the city centre gardens of Cape Town. Another statue of him riding his horse holding a map is located in Kimberly city.

A statue of him in the Harare city gardens was recently destroyed in 2001 after it was felt as inflammatory and is no more. His massive grave in Matopo Hills, near Bulawayo, is on a dominating hill that overlooks over 20 miles in every direction. The grave has not been tampered with and I last saw his grave when I was a Boy Scout aged about ten years. The last of the statues is in Kensington Palace Gardens and I saw it when I was in London aged 26 years. I saw all the other statues located in South Africa during my stay there, with the exception of the one in Kimberly. Surprisingly, no one has ever mentioned the wife or girlfriend of Cecil John Rhodes, for no one knows anything about her. He kept the 'information' close to his chest. However, he left a vast wealth in his will.[32] His Will funds 102 comprehensive scholarships to Oxford University in England every year at an annual cost of three million pounds for applicants mainly from the Commonwealth countries. The money is not showing any signs of exhaustion even after 109 years since his death!

Meanwhile, I was self-funding myself from my 'Mickey Mouse' savings that I had saved up while I was in London. My reserves were meant to cover all costs related to the educational undertakings. From my humble calculations, I should have survived for at least a year or so and then I would be skating on financial thin ice. I soon settled down and completed the registration process for the Masters in Medicine Degree in Anatomy, which was purely a research degree.

---

[32]http://en.wikipedia.org/wiki/Rhodes_Scholarship

My desire was to conduct a research project that would dovetail both my physiotherapy and anatomical experiences, and I craved to do something that would make a difference to the world we lived in. I decided to work on the anatomical abnormalities that make walking difficult for children with cerebral palsy. I had two co-supervisors, Professor Jennifer Jelsma, a professor of physiotherapy, who had once taught me while I was still at the University of Zimbabwe, and Professor Graham Louw. Professor Jelsma was a leading expert on determining which disability has greater impart than another disability. She would blush on being reminded that she once was the first runner up in the Miss University beauty pageant when she was an undergraduate. Her son, Braam Hanekom, always shook and rattled her comfort zone. Professor Jelsma would wake up to take a shower in order to go to work, only to find an immigrant busy in the shower, who could not utter a word of any of the languages she spoke. She frequently picked up and bailed out her son from the police station a dozen times for leading public protests. Braam helped start the 'People Against Suffering, Oppression and Poverty' charity[33], a hands-on non-profit organisation that defends the rights of asylum seekers, refugees and migrants in South Africa. Braam is a chip off the old block and his parents lived a similar life of supporting banned Africa National Congress activists during the apartheid years. He has won numerous national accolades and awards for being an exemplary youth. Valuable practical experience in human rights can be obtained by organising an internship with him!

My other co-supervisor, Professor Graham Louw, was a jovial man. He had trained as a veterinarian but had migrated to human anatomy some 20 years ago. He was well connected in the anatomy world and had contacts in almost every continent. He

---

[33]PASSOP, http://en.wikipedia.org/wiki/PASSOP

maintained a shaven head and an earring. We were of similar height and in some characteristic ways too. He never ever complained of my untidy desk, as his office too was usually scattered with all sorts of things on the four walls, on all the table surfaces, on all cupboards and even portions of the floor area.

It took me a good three months to develop a research proposal. The proposal highlighted what was known scientifically, what new knowledge could be added and how the study was to be carried out. After being given the nod by my two Professors, I applied and was given the ethical green light by the university. Ethical approval is now standard after some scientists conducted dubious research that harmed the unsuspecting participants. I had to use some specialised equipment, which measured the movement of a walking child and showed the movement on a computer. We had a torrid time trying to get access to the laboratory which was right under our departmental roof! I felt I was just outside the 'loop of circles' of those who could have access to the laboratory. Many meetings were held and a flurry of emails flew about but to no avail. It took over a year, from the time of getting ethical approval to realising that we would never ever get access to the laboratory. I had hoped to be finished with my dissertation by then and move forward with my career. I was also at the end of my financial steam too! Nevertheless, I have never made such good use of a year's time with alternative things as during that year.

Up to this time I did not have a single scientific publication to my name. The department of Human Biology had one of the best research track records that was envied across the entire University. It had a staff complement of 40 lecturers and 10 professors and annually notched up about 80 publications per year in rated journals. Such an environment left me so envious that I started cobbling together my most credible ideas I thought the world would like to hear about.

I started to dust off my previously completed studies and created new teaching approaches that I thought other university teachers across the world might be interested in. New research ideas were also initiated and cultivated. On average, it took me about five years to get a single journal publication and most of the different researches tended to run in parallel to each other. It took me about a year to conceptualise a good research idea that no one has ever worked on, two years to carry out the research, one year to write it up and a further year for the manuscript to pass through the journal review process. Even after the five years of hard work, my publication rate is 50% of manuscripts submitted, with which I am content.

My first manuscript submission was a three-dimension model of the heart and liver and was done by marking a gloved hand to resemble the odd shapes of the respective organs. I sent it to the *American Journal of Clinical Anatomy* and they declined it. I then went on to separate the manuscript into two parts, one with the model of the heart and the other with the liver. The liver manuscript was snatched up by the *Liver International Journal* within two days of it being sent.[34] The heart manuscript, which was far more elaborate and more scholarly, was declined by the *Europace Journal* and then by the *Lancet Medical Journal*. It finally found a home in the *British Journal of Cardiology* in May 2008.[35]

I showed Dr Warton the paper cadaver that I had invested over three hundred hours during the summer of 2004, whilst I was still in Zimbabwe. He suggested that I should modify it to a much simpler version. I then invested an additional six hundred hours

---

[34] http://onlinelibrary.wiley.com/doi/10.1111/j.1478-3231.2008.01709.x/abstract;jsessionid=3663A2DEDFF9E37A0BF24A8BA199456E.d01t02
[35] http://bjcardio.co.uk/2009/01/a-three-dimensional-anatomy-model-of-the-heart-organ-using-a-gloved-hand/

making the outlines of the shapes of muscles from wet cadavers, scanning the diagrams and fine tuning the diagram lines on a computer with Photoshop software. I incorporated the project into anatomy class practicals as a learning aid and it worked well. I submitted the concept to the *American Journal of Clinical Anatomy*, who accepted it after three further revisions.[36]

My dissertation for my BSc Physiotherapy degree was on finding the presence of the palmaris longus muscle at the front of the wrist among different people. Believe it or not, although 2% of Asians lack it, about 20% of Europeans do not have the muscle and the prevalence rate among Blacks was unknown. I found an absence rate of 2% on Blacks in Zimbabwe. I prepared a manuscript and also sent it to the *American Journal of Clinical Anatomy*, which accepted it after three revisions.[37] I prepared the research for my first ever academic conference, the 37th Annual Regional Conference of the Anatomical Society of Southern Africa, held in Magaliesburg in South Africa, which was entitled:

The clinical surface anatomy anomalies of the Palmaris Longus muscle in the Black African population of Zimbabwe and a proposed new testing technique.

My efforts landed me the 'SV Naidoo prize' for the Best Research Poster, one of the only four prizes on offer to the 85 research presentations.[38]

I co-authored a study which discovered an extra function of the palmaris longus muscle, of making the thumb stronger.[39] In a yet separate study of the palmaris longus, the assessment methods that are used during patient examinations to evaluate whether it is

---

[36]http://onlinelibrary.wiley.com/doi/10.1002/ca.20625/abstract
[37]http://onlinelibrary.wiley.com/doi/10.1002/ca.20751/abstract
[38]http://www.uct.ac.za/dailynews/archives/?id=6256
[39]http://onlinelibrary.wiley.com/doi/10.1002/ca.20961/abstract

present or not, were compared. I had proposed a new method I had invented for detecting the palmaris longus, called the 'Gangata Test', and it was one of the most effective tests. I sent the manuscript paper that compared the different tests to a few journals and they kept turning it down. It is a tough old world out there! The last study on the palmaris longus was a study by a BSc Honours Anatomy student that I co-supervised. It involved comparing the accuracy of manual methods to a method which used an ultrasound machine. She landed a distinction for her degree classification and is preparing the report to submit it to a medical journal.

On one of the days while I was at Jubilee church, I had a sort of a small 'eureka moment'. The Pastor was sharing a sermon on Isaiah 6, which describes an angel with six wings. One pair of wings covered its eyes, another pair covered the legs while the last pair of wings was used for flying. The description of the angel resembled a bone in the centre of the head called the 'sphenoid bone'. I had the pleasure of commissioning Luke Warton, a second year medical student who was the son of Dr Warton, to make a drawing of the heavenly scene. He took a well spent six months to make the drawing and the article was immediately and gladly accepted by the *British Journal of Oral and Medical Maxillofacial Surgery*.[40]

I had a passion for travelling and seeing the world. I frequently took breaks from my studies to see the world we lived in. Obviously the South African territory needed exploring and I founded the 'Liesbeeck Trotters' to mobilise university students to trot, not only the length and breadth of Cape Town, but the rest of South Africa and beyond to other countries of Southern

---

[40]http://www.sciencedirect.com/science/article/pii/S0266435610000975

Africa.[41] The most popular trips within Cape Town were visits to ice skating, visiting Robben Island, visiting penguins in Simon's Town and sea seals in Hout Bay. Three longer excursions were made during the university vacations. The first 600-mile round trip was by a group of eight students to Oudtshoorn, primarily to see the largest limestone cave in Africa; in total the caves stretched for over ten miles. Oudtshoorn had strong traditions of being the ostrich capital of the world for the last three hundred odd years or so. The bulk of the ostrich feathers that adorned the fancy hats of Victorian ladies, which had large plumages of ostriches sticking vertically upwards from their hats, came from this region. Fresh ostrich eggs were easily available for breakfast from the local nationwide 'Pick-n-Pay' supermarket in Oudtshoorn. A single ostrich egg is the equivalent of 24 chicken eggs!

The second 3000-mile round road trip to the nations of South Africa, Lesotho, Swaziland and Mozambique was undertaken by seven guys and passed through the 'Garden Route'.[42] The 'Garden Route' swept leisurely along the coastline from Cape Town to Durban through the greenest part of South Africa, while frequently peeping in to glance at the warm Indian Ocean for its entire length. After a respite in Durban, we headed westwards towards the famous Drakensburg Mountains, a UNESCO World Heritage Site. The Drakensburg Mountains are sandwiched between the tiny mountain kingdom of Lesotho and South Africa at the Sani Border Post. The Border Post probably has one of the steepest dusty roads in Africa and it became mandatory for travellers to have a four-wheeled vehicle in order to have their passports stamped. The steep Sani Border Post has preserved one of the most untouched parts of Africa, eastern Lesotho. Eastern

---

[41]http://www.uct.ac.za/print/mondaypaper/archives/?id=6715 and
http://www.uct.ac.za/print/mondaypaper/archives/?id=6554)
[42] The route is illustrated on the map on page 104

Lesotho has hundreds of mountains washed throughout the year by thousands of perennial rivers. Indeed, water is the largest export of Lesotho to South African cities like Johannesburg. We re-entered South Africa from Lesotho on our way to yet another kingdom, the Kingdom of Swaziland, and lastly made a one-day visit to Mozambique.

The last and most demanding trip was a four-week '6000-mile trip' from the southern tip of Africa to the halfway line across the African continent along the Equator. It snaked through South Africa, Zimbabwe, Mozambique, Malawi, Tanzania, Zanzibar, Zambia, back to Victoria Falls in Zimbabwe and returned home to South Africa.[43] We had to get visas, have prophylactic vaccinations and pack portable travelling gadgets and equipment, like sleeping bags and tents, into huge backpacks. My backpack weighed almost fifty pounds! We had to change mobile sim cards of different countries, like changing socks, in order to get the best phone tariffs! The three most magical moments were in Malawi, Zanzibar and Victoria Falls. The three days on the seventy-year old Ilala ferry, while it grunted through the largest fresh water lake in the world, Lake Malawi, felt so exotic. We walked on the four-hundred-year-old exceptionally narrow streets of Stone town, capital of Zanzibar, another UNESCO World Heritage Site. The untouched and unconstructed white beaches of Zanzibar were licked by the warm clear waters of the Indian Ocean. It was magical. Victoria Falls is a must for every earthling. The Victoria Falls are literally one mile wide and the waters drop for over 140 yards in a slow motion manner. A minimum of two days is required to make a decent view of the falls. The falls make the sound of the rumblings of a hundred simultaneous trains.

---

[43] The route is illustrated on the map on page[104]

As might be expected of such ambitious expeditions into unfamiliar territory, there were twists and turns. One unpredictable turn was on the outbound leg of the trip. We were on a nearly full bus that took us through three countries and four border posts in fourteen hours. The ZUPCO bus left Harare in Zimbabwe at nine o'clock in the morning, some two hours later than it should have left. No one was really bothered and everyone was quite relaxed about it. It was supposed to arrive in the capital of Malawi, Blantyre, at 7p.m. in the evening, but by nine in the evening, we still had not entered Malawi. On reaching the Mozambique Border Post shortly after 8p.m., the passports of the entire bus were rapidly cleared and we arrived at the Malawi Border in the nick of time—some five minutes before nine o'clock. They closed at nine o'clock!

I was among the first who rushed to the Malawi Immigration Office. A 'cheeky immigration official' took one long look at us and, much to our horror, closed shop with some five minutes of official time remaining. I guess he knew he needed at least half an hour to properly check the passports and bags for the whole bus. Perhaps his boss did not pay him overtime! The price was high. People had to sleep in the bus in which they had spent the whole fourteen hours travelling. We had fortunately packed tents into our backpacks and slept well in them. The only downside was that one of our co-travellers forgot his shoes outside the tent, to avoid soiling his tent, and the night rain left them soaking wet by the morning. The shoes he wore were the only shoes he had because he wanted to lighten his backpack load! The 'cheeky immigration officer' probably slept well and in the morning cleared our grumpier bus commuters.

The holiday was filled with other adventures and at the end of them I returned to Cape Town to continue with my research projects.

Chapter 13

Reloading My Research Passions in South Africa

A FTER ALMOST A FULL YEAR of dilly dallying, my supervisors and I decided to knock out the component of my study needing the Gait laboratory and replace it with something else. I liaised with the three schools in Cape Town, which were almost exclusively for children with disabilities, in order to contact the parents and guardians for permission. I got started after a couple of weeks of running in circles to get the consent forms signed. I collected the various complex measurements of the legs of children with cerebral palsy. I wanted to find out what was causing them to use so much energy in walking. They were using six times more energy than children developing normally, i.e. if you walk ten metres to the kitchen and back, they would have walked the distance six-fold. The main findings of the study were that weak calf muscles greatly and disproportionally increased the energy cost of walking. The study was the first to discover that children with cerebral palsy who were affected in both knees tended to have a triad syndrome of short hamstring muscles, walking with bent knees and weak muscles that straighten the knees.

After scribbling through a hundred drafts or so, my two professors finally gave me the nod to formally submit the dissertation to the University of Cape Town for marking. The research was examined by other professors abroad over a period of three months. The first report was full of praise and he recommended a distinction and the second professor felt it was just between good and average, but not really outstanding. The University of Cape Town examinations board decided on just a pass mark for the dissertation. Oh, what a big hug Professor Jelsma gave me, and Professor Louw had a big smile for the rest of the week!

In the winter of 2008, an entirely unexpected hell broke loose in South Africa.[44] The homes and houses of non-South African Africans were razed to the ground by infernos led by Black South African armed mobs with sticks and other weapons. It started in the township of Alexandra in Johannesburg. The Black South African mobs moved from street to street, witch-hunting for any Africans without a South African accent to lynch. The Africans, who were fairly easy to spot for they were generally taller and darker than the Black South Africans counterparts, were blamed for taking away local jobs, housing and for cranking up crime in the country. The Somali community, who had a relatively low educational inclination and had all but given up any real chance of getting formal jobs, had thriving small convenience grocery shops scattered among the townships. Most of the shops were looted and razed to the ground after the owners fled with their dear lives. The mayhem eventually spread to all the main cities in South Africa within about two weeks and the Governments of African countries moved quickly. Mozambique charted a number of trains to get their citizens back home, as did Zimbabwe, Malawi, Zambia, Namibia and other countries in providing transport for their nationals.

Most of the African leaders painfully remembered the time when they gave logistical, moral, financial and exile support to the Black South African politicians during the apartheid years. As

---

[44]http://en.wikipedia.org/wiki/Xenophobia_in_South_Africa#May_2008_riots

for us, we sought to the find the meaning of the opening lines of the South African national anthem which went 'God bless Africa'. South Africa had had the whole-hearted support from the rest of Africa of hosting the first ever Football World Cup on African soil and Africans were struggling to come to terms with whether they would be welcome to come and watch the football matches. In the aftermath of the xenophobia, it so happened that one third of those killed were actually Black South Africans who were from minor tribes![45] There was a huge humanitarian programme launched by charities and the South African Government to deal with the hundreds of thousands of displaced people. A large number of Black South Africans chipped in making meals and providing humanitarian assistance. Although the universities were insulated from the xenophobia, we thereafter kept the Black residential areas at arm's length.

My greatest sense of contributing to South Africa came from the research supervisory work I did while I was at the University of Cape Town. A student I co-supervised was selected to present orally his research on the palmaris longus muscle on a Research Day of the Medical School. He was one of the six oral presentations allowed that year from all the undergraduates at the medical school. Another student studied for her BSc Honours in Anatomy and was awarded a distinction degree class for work on using ultrasound to find the palmaris longus muscle.

The two pairs of ladies whose research I co-supervised appeared in the 2010 university annual alumni magazine as an encouragement to Black women that they can pursue and succeed in carrying out research at a high international level.[46] The first pair of young ladies studying medicine, Ms Thandeka Ngcongo and Ms Mitchell Bontle, published their work in the *American*

---

[45]http://en.wikipedia.org/wiki/Xenophobia_in_South_Africa
[46]http://www.alumninews.uct.ac.za/downloads/uctnews_2010.pdf

Journal of Clinical Anatomy for work on the palmaris longus. They determined the rate of absence among the Cape Coloureds and was the first ever study to do so. About 50% of Cape Town is a mixed race.[47] The second pair of two medical students, Ms Princess Akol and Ms Phatheka Ntaba, sought to find the source of cadavers in most African countries. We had realised that the sources of cadavers in Africa have been unknown while most of the cadavers used in developed countries are donated. Medical schools across the world require cadavers to train medical doctors how the body is organised. The human body is incredibly complex and has over 200 differently shaped bones and over 600 separate muscles. It is far better for a training doctor to practice surgery on cadavers than to have their very first surgery on someone's aunt or mother.

Their results were that most of the medical schools in Africa were using unclaimed bodies from hospitals and prisons, who were typically of poor males detached from their families. The only country with a meaningful number of donations was South Africa. They found that most of the donations in South Africa could be traced to newspaper and radio requests for dead human bodies by Professor Emeritus Phillip Tobias in the late 1950's and at least 6 000 donations have since been made to two of the South African medical schools. Of almost all cases in Africa, most of the donations were by the White and Coloured community. The non-donation of cadavers by Blacks was attributed to strong cultural beliefs and the lack of awareness of body donation programmes. This led to African countries with much lower populations of White and Coloured communities solely relying on unclaimed bodies. They also found that the use of unclaimed bodies in developed countries have been discouraged because it violates the wishes of the cadavers. The

---

[47]http://onlinelibrary.wiley.com/doi/10.1002/ca.20961/abstract

research appeared in the *American Journal of Anatomical Sciences Education*.[48] The one impression that was seared onto our minds, as we were working on the research, was the thought that "some people were so generous that death is not enough to stop their generosity". Anyone interested in donating their cadaver for the training of medical doctors should contact their nearest university with a medical school or their nearest doctor.

The research work on cadavers has since influenced and been cited by academics in Africa, Asia and the USA.[49] I dropped Phatheka and Princess an email to let them know how appreciated their work has been. They replied with the following emails expressing profound surprise:

Email from Miss PhathekaNtaba:

Re: A follow-up study of sources of cadavers in Africa

From: Phatheka NTABA <NTBPHA001@uct.ac.za>
*   Tuesday, 17 May 2011, 11:54*

To: Hope Gangata<hopegata@yahoo.co.uk>

Hey Hope

---

[48]http://onlinelibrary.wiley.com/doi/10.1002/ase.157/abstract
[49]Akinola OB. Formal body bequest program in Nigerian medical schools: When do we start?
AnatSci Educ. 2011 Jul;4(4):239-42. doi: 10.1002/ase.226. Epub 2011 May 12.
Cornwall J.The diverse utility of wet prosections and plastinated specimens in teaching gross anatomy in New Zealand.AnatSci Educ. 2011 Jul 22. doi: 10.1002/ase.245. [Epub ahead of print]
Jones DG, Whitaker MI. Anatomy's use of unclaimed bodies: Reasons Against Continued Dependence on an Ethically Dubious Practice. Clin Anat. 2011 Jul 28. doi: 10.1002/ca.21223. [Epub ahead of print]
Ballala K, Shetty A, Malpe SB. Knowledge, attitude, and practices regarding whole body donation among medical professionals in a hospital in India.AnatSci Educ. 2011 May 4(3):142-50. doi: 10.1002/ase.220. Epub 2011 May 5.

I am so humbled right now, it's not even funny!!!
Thanks for letting us know.
You're the best!
Phatheka

Email from Miss Princess Akol:

Re: A follow-up study of sources of cadavers in Africa

From: *Princess AKOL <aklpri001@uct.ac.za>*
          Tuesday, 17 May 2011, 15:20

To: *hopegata@yahoo.co.uk*

Hi Hope

It has been quite a while, I'm well. I trust work and life that side is treating you good?

It's encouraging & enlightening to know that all that work could inspire someone.

Keep well.

Regards,
Princess

Work on the palmaris longus muscle[50] and other papers[51] have also received citations by numerous other medical researchers.

---

[50]Erić M, Koprivčić I, Vučinić N, Radić R, Krivokuća D, Lekšan I, Selthofer R. Prevalence of the palmaris longus in relation to the hand dominance. SurgRadiol Anat. 2011 Aug;33(6):481-4. Epub 2010 Nov 24.

K. Devi Sankar, P. SharmilaBhanu, and Susan P. John.Incidence of agenesis of palmaris longus in the Andhra population of India. Indian J Plast Surg. 2011 Jan-Apr; 44(1): 134–138.

Although the stellar status of science based industries and science in universities in South Africa is renown throughout Africa, the mass secondary and high school teaching of science and mathematics has room for improvement. My humble advice to the Ministry of Education of South Africa is perhaps to tweak, restructure or replace the Matriculation examination system. South Africa has neither O-levels, the eleventh year of schooling,

Sater MS, Dharap AS, Abu-Hijleh MF.The prevalence of absence of the palmaris longus muscle in the Bahraini population.Clin Anat. 2010 Nov;23(8):956-61.
S. Oladipo Gabriel, C. Didia Blessing & A. Ugboma : Frequency Of Agenesis Of The Palmaris Longus Muscle In Nigerians. The Internet Journal of Biological Anthropology. 2009 Volume 3 Number
M Deniz. 2011. The prevalence and familial tendency of absence of the palmaris longus muscle in Turkish population. Pakistan Journal of Medical Sciences

[51]Venail F, Deveze A, Lallemant B, Guevara N, Mondain M. Enhancement of temporal bone anatomy learning with computer 3D rendered imaging software. Med Teach. 2010;32(7):e282-8.
Chan LK, Cheng MM. An analysis of the educational value of low-fidelity anatomy models as external representations. AnatSci Educ. 2011 Jul 8. doi: 10.1002/ase.239. [Epub ahead of print]
McCulloch C, Marango SP, Friedman ES, Laitman JT. Living AnatoME: Teaching and learning musculoskeletal anatomy through yoga and pilates. AnatSci Educ. 2010 Nov-Dec;3(6):279-86. doi: 10.1002/ase.181. Epub 2010 Oct 1.
Hayes JA, Ivanusic JJ, le Roux CM, Hatzopoulos K, Gonsalvez D, Hong S, Durward C. Collaborative development of anatomy workshops for medical and dental students inCambodia. AnatSci Educ. 2011 Jun 27. doi: 10.1002/ase.238. [Epub ahead of print]
Inuwa IM, Al Rawahy M, Taranikanti V, Habbal O. Anatomy "steeplechase" online: necessity sometimes is the catalyst for innovation. AnatSci Educ. 2011 Mar-Apr;4(2):115-8. doi: 10.1002/ase.188. Epub 2010 Dec 2.
Hiz Ö, Ediz L , Ceylan MF, Gezici E, Gülcü E, Erden M. 2011. Prevalence of the absence of palmaris longus muscle assessed by a new examination test (Hiz-Ediz Test) in the population residing in the area of Van, Turkey. Journal of Clinical and Experimental Investigations; 2 (3): 254-259
Inuwa IM, Taranikanti V, Al-Rawahy M, Habbal O. 2011. Anatomy practical examinations: How does student performance on computerized evaluation compare with the traditional format? AnatSci Educ. Sep 13. doi: 10.1002/ase.254. [Epub ahead of print]

nor A-levels as the thirteenth year of schooling. Instead, it has the Matriculation examination in the twelve year in which pupils are expected to sit examinations in a minimum of six subjects that are at AS-level,[52] with some brave ones taking up to ten subjects. The system kills two birds with one stone. Students who achieve over 40% across the six subjects are confirmed the 'Higher Standard Grade' (the AS-level equivalent), while those who nudge the 33% mark per subject across six subjects are accorded the 'Standard Grade' (the O-level equivalent).

The whole tragedy of the system is that the exceptionally fragile learning of science and mathematics has been overstretched. A first-year medical or engineering university student unfortunately receives the same amount of science education as a humanity or commercial university first year by the time they leave high school. Furthermore, science education is relatively more expensive to run than humanities or commercials. Science education requires a science laboratory equipped with chemicals and various apparatus such as pipettes and beakers. The financial and manpower resources for science have become so stretched that science practicals are no longer compulsory across the country. Indeed, physics, chemistry or biology matriculation practical examinations have also been pruned out. Worse still, the science passion in some of the pupils is not matched with quality time from the best science teachers. The science teachers spend an inordinate amount of time on students that have no interest at all in taking on a science career.

Science and mathematics are very delicate subjects to learn and get progressively more complicated year by year. The work of one year in science or mathematics is more essential for the understanding of the sequential learning for the following year

---

[52]An AS-level subject is the first year of the two-year 'A-level' subject.

than in humanities. Skipping two years' work in mathematics certainly leads to a learning brick wall when you want to continue following the scribbling of mathematics on the blackboard two years later. History, as an example of humanities, will not be as much affected. The two-year gap will require competent and experienced mathematics and science teachers who are proficient enough to diagnose the learning potholes and fill them satisfactorily to smooth the road enough for the next mathematical lesson.

There are two separate one-way valves bleeding the scientific manpower from South Africa—the internal valve and the migratory valve. Retaining science and mathematics teachers is an equally slippery slope and is the internal one-way valve. A science graduate can switch to a different field, like commercials, with relatively more ease. Graduates from humanities and commercials, however, cannot switch to science-related professions at the drop of a hat, like being a medical doctor, engineer or science teacher. The high analytical skills among science graduates have become so much sought after by the banking industry and other industries looking for applicants for trainee managers. The science graduates of South Africa are a highly sought after group abroad, with South African nurses, doctors and science teachers being good examples. South African nurses are the second largest nationality working in the United Kingdom, while 37% of all the South African doctors are working abroad.[53] South African doctors have been preferred in English speaking Western countries because "they were trained well, spoke English fluently, and were White".[54] South Africa is fighting with one hand tied behind its back through red tape. It signed a pact to ban any nurse or doctor from the regional block of neighbouring countries from working in South Africa,

---

[53]http://www.twnside.org.sg/title2/gtrends99.htm
[54]http://www.bmj.com/content/310/6990/1307.full

ensuring a one-way migratory valve. The science manpower shortages are glaringly evident from the jobs that can elicit a work permit in South Africa for foreign workers. All but one of the job professions listed are science-related careers, like engineers, geologists and statisticians![55]

The buck was obviously passed to the universities to sort out. The South African universities coined four-year degree courses that are three years in duration in most countries, in a bid to deal with the problem. The four-year degree models are struggling to cope with the deficits on mathematics and science in some of the students. Thus most of the South African universities have bent backwards to create five-year degree programs for what should be taught in three years. Obviously it is so much more expensive to teach students at university, something that should have been taught during high school and is not sustainable.

It might be beneficial for the country as a whole if the architects of science education had a rethink on the matriculation system. Input from the Vice Chancellors of South African universities to the educational architects would be beneficial. South Africa is one of the leading countries and the pride of Africa in scientific expertise. Sadly that advantage has not translated in South Africa by exporting science-related manpower to the other African countries. Re-crafting the science high school education may unlock and blossom greater numbers of the youth undertaking a passionate full career in the sciences. South Africa is one of the few African countries lucky enough to afford paying its teachers salaries of between $US1000 and $US2500 per month. Maximizing the relatively large funds allocated to education should assist in propelling South Africa into the future.

---

[55] http://www.safis.co.il/site/wp-content/uploads/2010/01/Permits.pdf

I left South Africa before it hosted the first ever World Cup tournament on African soil in 2010. I had innocently sent the University of Cape Town a message saying, 'Please do Africa proud by hosting the tournament well.' The message somehow reached the desk of the Vice Chancellor of the university, Dr Max Price, and he acknowledged it in the Alumni News magazine of 2010 and confirmed that it was hosted rather too well.[56]

---

[56]http://www.alumninews.uct.ac.za/report-back/vc-foreword/

Chapter 14

Inflation Years

I HAVE LIVED THROUGH very unpredictable and trying times. The reserve bank of Zimbabwe went on an unprecedented printing spree from 2004 to 2009 and produced the second worst inflation in the history of the world, with Hungary in 1946 getting the trophy. The Zimbabwean dollar was highly valued at US$1.50 when it was introduced in 1980 to replace the Rhodesian dollar, and fell from grace to be the most worthless currency by late 2008. Gideon Gono, the Governor of the Reserve Bank of Zimbabwe from 2003 to date in 2012, wrote a book hilariously called the *Zimbabwe's Casino Economy* in 2008.

Gono introduced four waves of currency notes in response to a paralysed economy and restless trade unions. The first wave was a stop gap measure set of 'bearer's cheques' that were meant to operate as travellers' cheques. The 'bearer's cheques' were printed in a huff on one side of the old $Zim50 notes while on the other side the features of the old $Zim50 could still be seen. They were printed in flavours of $Zim5000 to $Zim100 000 and turned us into gentlemen once again: we could now carry about money that could easily fit into a wallet. In 2005 a pie was $Zim15000 and the highest old note before the 'bearer's cheques' was $Zim50. Thus, a pie needed a humongous pile of three hundred notes of $Zim50 notes.

In the 80's, notice of a price hike was usually given a decent two months ahead of the intended price hike. The notice gave people enough time to regroup and explore other product or service substitutes. In time, the notice period wilted to just a few days until it became virtually a few hours, as in 2004, when petrol prices were hiked 'with effect from midnight'. The pace of the inflation gathered more speed, until about 2006 when the notices for price hikes vanished altogether. Prices were silently notched up overnight while we slept. It saved many companies the humiliation of apologising for yet another round of price hikes within a month and probably saved them some advertising costs also. Soon enough, we all got a rude awakening when prices doubled or trebled each time we wanted to restock our grocery supplies.

The cash would not even fit into a handbag, let alone a gentleman's wallet. The 'bearer's cheques' were intentionally released in drips and were extremely difficult to come across because of the Reserve Bank, banks in general or by business tycoons. The Reserve Bank of Zimbabwe literally drip fed the new notes into the banks, which in turn released the notes through the back doors. The few 'bearer's cheques' that reached the public suffered a one-way traffic route to the private cash vaults of shop owners, transport companies and industrialists. Cash purchases were rewarded with a discount of 10% to 20% of the marked price. This was around the time I relocated from Zimbabwe to London in early 2005.

The printing of the bank notes went on and on like a radio on a new battery. The inflation rate exceeded 1000% per year in 2006 and pies were priced in millions of dollars. The Governor slashed three zeros from notes and issued a second family of notes in August of 2006. It worked wonders for a couple of months before things were back to square one, with pies costing millions again by January of 2007. In January 2008, the same pies were literally costing tens of billions of dollars. The Governor chopped off as many zeros as he could for a second time and issued a redenominated Zimbabwean dollar in August of 2008, amputating ten zeros in the process! The new one Zimbabwean dollar was worth ten billion of its preceding currency after its issuance by the Reserve Bank of Zimbabwe. Pies cost a dollar or two for a few days once more. By Christmas of 2008 pies were costing trillions of dollars once again. Yet another local currency massage was given in February of 2009 and twelve zeros were written off from the Zimbabwean dollar. It was too late, almost everyone had lost faith in the currency and even the government railways and the Post Office no longer accepted the local currency. On 12 April 2009, the Government of Zimbabwe finally conceded defeat of the Zimbabwean dollar and accepted the formal use of the United States dollar. Inflation dropped to less than 1% overnight and has hardly exceeded that figure to date in 2012.

The Government tried all sorts of gears to combat inflation and even officially declared inflation illegal in 2007 without resolving its economic drivers. Any mortal who dared to notch up prices after a certain date was duly arrested. This policy did not work and brought more confusion into an already unpredictable economic setting. The policy led to more frustration and unbelievable levels of secrecy in the conduct of day-to-day business. The banning of the use of foreign currency, which started in 1980, was eventually lifted in January of 2009. Money supply was choked off by restricting withdrawals to a whiff but this badly backfired when almost everyone stopped depositing money into banks. The price of pies in the shops had to be adjusted several times a day during the worst period. It was noted that a certain fellow who ordered a second cup of tea was charged a higher price than for his first cup.

"Order and get the two cups delivered simultaneously if you want the same price," grunted the waiter.

Two years after the end of inflation in 2011, the Governor Gideon Gono pleaded with parliament and the Ministry of Finance to restart printing a national currency. They flatly refused as their memories were still too fresh. For the first time since Independence in 1980, the Ministry of Finance was led by the opposition party, the Movement of Democratic Congress (MDC). The parliament was evenly split between Mugabe's ZANU PF and the MDC. An agreement to form a government of national unity was signed into law in September 2008 by the three political parties.

The biggest losers were those with long term savings and pensioners who were no longer working. Their monthly pensions diminished in value and ended up being less than the cost of a postage stamp. This made the monthly pension not even worth collecting. These pensioners had bought large bungalow houses in Harare for about $Zim20 000 at the time of Independence in 1980. A typical bungalow house bought then had four bedrooms and a swimming pool on a four-acre piece of land. And now, to buy a single brick was setting you back a couple of million dollars! The plight of British pensioners became so desperate that the British High Commissioner in Zimbabwe arranged the total repatriation of between 500 and 1500 frail elderly persons over the age of 70 years back to England, as long as they could prove their citizenship by ancestry. The British government provided flights, housing and financial support to all those who took up the offer.[57]

---

[57]http://www.huffingtonpost.com/2009/06/05/zimbabwe-whites-flown-bac_n_211858.html and
http://www.telegraph.co.uk/news/worldnews/africaandindianocean/zimbabwe/5394171/Zimbabwes-destitute-Britons-to-be-repatriated.html

The working class like myself somehow fared relatively better above the inflation cloud by literally inflating back the cost of our services. I recalibrated upwards the fees I charged for privately teaching anatomy. The supply and demand factors were in our favour as science graduates. There was hardly any other person who had specialised in anatomy and had the time to teach anatomy privately. There was a similar high demand for physiotherapists around the country too and their salaries were primed up and upgraded after every couple of months.

There was the sad case of a hard working corn farmer who sold his bumper harvest of corn at good market prices. He did not trust the banks with his money and it was for good reason. The banks in Zimbabwe then were a nuisance and made one queue for hours to get a whiff of the money one demanded. The monetary policy then was to choke off inflation by strangulating the money supply from the banks. And so the farmer simply hid his stash of cash under his bed for a year until the next farming season. He would gleefully check his treasure every morning when he woke up and pull out a genuine smile. He finally unleashed his fortune when it came to the next planting season, in order to buy seeds and fertiliser. He was immediately horrified to discover that his accumulated treasure had been wilted by inflation so severely that it could not even buy him a teaspoon of seed.

Inflation of A-level grades in England is equally worrying. All inflated things have a cosy bubble within, in which an appetite for getting even more inflated exists. The bubble has an awesome 'feel good' sense of satisfaction because it creates an appearance of progress. We enjoyed having more and more zeros on our payslips while we were in Zimbabwe for a while. For the last 29 years, the proportion of A-level grades with A-grades has been notching up steadily on a yearly basis. Twenty years ago only 9% of A-level candidates achieved A-grades but that has now shot up to 27% of all candidates scoring an A-grade. The then C-grade is now the equivalent of the current A-grade.[58] There were so many A-grades by 2009 that a new A*-grade was introduced so as to clear the muddied waters and enable universities to identify the best students. The A*-grade may soon lose its punch at the current rate of grade inflation. A new A**-grade may soon be required and within nine years it will be impossible for anyone to fail A-levels.[59] The A*-and A-grades are appearing against a reality that the United Kingdom is falling on world rankings on literacy and numeracy tables.[60]

Recent new entrants to university in the United Kingdom are weaker on critical reading, writing arguments and grammar skills.[61] Emeritus professor at Buckingham University, John Marks, examined O-level mathematics questions given over the last 50 years, and noted in an unflattering report that algebra and geometry were being replaced with mere arithmetic, and questions were becoming less demanding.[62] Comparable qualifications such as the International Baccalaureate have gained in status at the expense of A-levels and the International Baccalaureate is now worth five A-levels lumped together, instead of the original three A-levels.[63]

It is worth noting that the number of university places are finite and are offered on a competitive basis to the very best students.

---

[58]http://www.telegraph.co.uk/comment/6063012/A-level-results-grade-inflation-is-just-a-cruel-confidence-trick.html and
http://www.bbc.co.uk/news/education-14558490
http://www.telegraph.co.uk/comment/6063012/A-level-results-grade-inflation-is-just-a-cruel-confidence-trick.html
[60]http://www.oecd.org/dataoecd/34/60/46619703.pdf
[61]http://www.educationmatters.ie/?p=393
[62]http://www.reform.co.uk/Research/Education/EducationArticles/tabid/110/smid/378/ArticleID/621/reftab/71/t/The%20value%20of%20mathematics/Default.aspx
[63]http://www.independent.co.uk/news/education/schools/international-baccalaureate-why-the-broad-ib-beats-alevels-395262.html

Having a certain grade will not guarantee a place. Inflation of the A-level results simply notches up the entry requirements for degree programmes. Indeed, the University of Cambridge has sadly turned down 5817 applicants in 2011 who had three straight A-grades at A-level and is now requiring the new A*-grades.[64] The philosophy of 'medals for everyone' is producing a lot of winners but not translating them into champions. It is not the fault of students at all as they still put in the seriousness that their predecessors put in. Competing institutions that offer A-level examinations have been blamed for loosening the standards because they became popular for offering schools and pupils an easier way of achieving high grades for university. There is hardly any grade inflation in Scotland where there exists just one awarding institution.[65] Some have put the blame of grade inflation in United Kingdom on the switching from norm referenced marking to criterion referencing marking for both O-levels and A-level in 1986. Norm referenced marking allocates A-grades to say the top 5% of examination candidates. On the other hand, criterion referencing marking system allocates and awards A-grades for everyone who has passed a certain percentage mark deemed to be enough work to get an A-grade, of say 60%, irrespective of how many pupils get above 60%. Successive Governments in the United Kingdom are said to have turned a blind eye to the grade inflation to make it seem like the school performances have improved on their watch.

While for some of us the average performance is all we want to settle for, for those who want to raise their aspirations, a higher standard is the key. It is important to embed a theme of competiveness on your work. Hours simply have to be ploughed into any career to remain competitive and it will be those very

---

[64]http://www.dailymail.co.uk/news/article-1269635/Cambridge-rejects-5-800-straight-A-pupils.html
[65]http://fullfact.org/factchecks/grade_inflation_rising_results_falling_standards-1538

hours that will give that extra edge that the college or job interview selectors will chase after in applications. Add an extra subject if you can and take on a 'Duke of Edinburgh' certificate during your high schooling to fortify your CV if you can. We have an idiomatic saying in Zimbabwe which says "no one knows what the pig ate to make it fat". For everything that you send an application for, you need to stand shoulders above the other applicants. Smiling and charming your way through the interview will not give you a leg against the other applicants. Deeper roots will be required. I topped up a couple more extra O-level sciences to my normal load of eight subjects during a time when I moved houses five times to live in different households over a space of one year. I added an extra A-level subject of Further Mathematics when I was heavily involved as part of the leadership of Scripture Union. The leaders had an awful reputation of being academic insulators for the four preceding straight years. I beefed up my undergraduate physiotherapy degree with an anatomy undergraduate degree to become the first of a handful of Zimbabwean anatomists to come from a physiotherapy background. I finished my Masters in Anatomy in a foreign country at a time of unprecedented inflation in Zimbabwe. I have just finished my second masters, Masters of Arts in Higher Education Practice, just to stay ahead of the game. I cannot wait to restart my delayed PhD in early 2012 after putting it on hold in 2009.

Chapter 15

The Sad Passing Away of Senior Medical Teachers of Zimbabwe

THE YEAR OF 2007 WAS THE SADDEST in the history of the medical school of the University of Zimbabwe. The medical teachers who passed away that year were not replaced by either expatriates, as Zimbabwe was at the most painful part of the rampant inflation, nor by the locals. It would require persons with at least 30 years of postgraduate medical teaching experience to replace each of these men. The shoes of these men are still unfilled to this very day!

It was with great sadness that I learnt that most of my learned teachers and professors at the medical school at the University of Zimbabwe passed away, one after another, at a time when I was moving towards being a teacher at a medical school. It all happened in the space of a year or so. The first to pass away was Professor DM Katzarski. He was a Bulgarian anatomist who had taken a keen interest in teaching embryology, the study of the developing unborn baby. He had taught embryology and gross anatomy at the University of Zimbabwe for over two decades and was in a green old age. He must have been in his late 80's and had never had a fall out with any of the lecturers or students, so good natured was he.

Professor Katzarski was a very intelligent lecturer but somehow he could not face up to his demons. He did not overcome his cyberphobia (fear of computers), and avoided learning how to use the basic features of a computer. He claimed "it was too complicated". He used to write to his family in Bulgaria and his letter took over three weeks to get there. By the time he got their reply, two months had gone by. It finally dawned on him that email was the way to go after his daughter convinced him. He would write a letter on paper, ask the anatomy secretary to open a new email account and to send the letter on his behalf. The secretary would log on to his email account once in a while, to check for new emails and kindly print the reply emails for him and put them into his normal letter box marked with his name. He would then archive the printed emails in a filing cabinet after reading them. Professor Katzarski was the only lecturer who did not have a computer in his office.

The second professor was Professor Reid Harris, probably from the United Kingdom. He had taught clinical medicine for over a decade at the University of Zimbabwe. I did not know him personally but nevertheless felt the loss. The next loss was a Dr Muchenagumbo, who was a consultant neurosurgeon and one of less than ten in the country. He was heavily involved in teaching clinical neurosurgery in ward rounds. Despite his tangible pride, he really enjoyed teaching and he would 'hi five' any of us in his ward round who guessed the diagnosis right. I am told he spent his last days doing his ward rounds, from a wheelchair. Neurosurgery was his life.

The next national loss was the passing away of Professor Laurence Francis Levy (1921-2007, MRCS 1945; FRCS 1955; MB BS London 1948; MSc New York 1954; LRCP 1945; FRCS Edin 1982; FACS) in May 2007. He was the 'first neurosurgeon in Sub-Saharan Africa'.[66] Professor Levy was the consultant neurosurgeon for the Salisbury Group of Hospitals (Rhodesia) since1956. His services extended as far as the Congo, Tanzania and Mozambique.[67] He was a Professor of Surgery and his hallmark contribution to surgery was the design of the 'Harare shunt' to drain excess fluid from the brains of children with hydrocephalus, a condition where water accumulates in the brain. The Harare shunt used a normal $US5 nasogastric tube to replace the over-rated $US230 Hakim-Codman tube.[68] The nasogastric tube had a slit lower end and had 'no pump or ant siphon mechanism' and worked remarkably well. The Harare shunt has since been adopted in many countries in Africa and other developing countries, and has had satisfactory long term effects.

Levy was also the Head of the Department of Anatomy at the University of Zimbabwe from the 1970s and until he retired in 2006. Professor Levy believed in us. It was during his leadership at the Department of Anatomy that the department allowed me to be the first Zimbabwean from the Physiotherapy field to study the BSc (Intercalated) Honours in Human Anatomy degree in 2000. It was also during the time that he was the Head of the Department of Anatomy, that I rose from being an applicant to the University of Zimbabwe for the BSc Physiotherapy degree programme to a student of Physiotherapy, then a student of anatomy, followed by being an anatomy Demonstrator. I became a supervisor of a team of dissectors of anatomy specimens, an Anatomy Teaching Assistant, an Anatomy Junior Lecturer and finally a Course Convener for the Anatomy course studied by the Physiotherapy and Occupational Therapy undergraduate degree programmes. All this happened in a space of six years. I doubt

[66]http://livesonline.rcseng.ac.uk/biogs/E001133b.htm
[67]http://www.bioline.org.br/request?js07032
[68]http://www.springerlink.com/content/tdbkkxfj16mewq73/fulltext.pdf

whether my 'two minute chats' would still get me a job in the department of Anatomy anymore, now that he is gone.

I should note that during all the years that I was with him, I had never seen him wearing gloves in the dissecting laboratory. He preferred using his bare hands. Professor Levy was my academic mentor and my research supervisor for the thesis entitled:

> *The non-rarity of herniated discs in the indigenous population of Zimbabwe: A cadaveric and epidemio logical study.* BSc Hons Hum Anat Thesis, University of Zimbabwe. June 2001.

Lawrence was well respected by the staff and students in the department, the university fraternity and even at the four referral hospitals. He used to bring a large consignment of mulberries from his farm to refresh the staff at the department.

The high calibre of medical graduates from the University of Zimbabwe honestly frightened him because they were so good that the First World countries were poaching the few doctors we struggled to produce. The First World countries had not shown any seriousness in increasing the training and retention of their local health staff. Well, to prevent the First World countries from "fishing from the same pond", he proposed in the *British Medical Journal* in 2003 reconfiguring the Zimbabwean curriculums to make it internationally incompatible, so as to save medical staff from going away.[69] With that being said, I will not forget that it was on my first ever trip to England for an anatomy interview at the University of East Anglia, that he gave me a £20 note from his own pocket. Quite a down-to-earth man he was. 'Sekuru' will be missed.[70]

---

[69] http://www.bmj.com/content/327/7407/Reviews.full.pdf
[70] 'Sekuru' is vernacular for grandpa.

My nearest loss was the death of Dr Isidore Pazvakavambwa. He was an albino and was born into a lowly rural family. He defied the odds and became the country's only paediatric cardiologist, who treated heart conditions of babies, and was a consultant at all the four hospitals in Harare, the capital city. He was instrumental in pushing the Government to have children less than five years of age to be treated for free in Government hospitals. He was the closest to me of all the medical teachers who had passed away because we attended the same church, Faith Ministries, and he was one of my mentors. I miss the wise words he gave at men's fellowship meetings. He passed away a few weeks after my journal article was accepted into the *British Journal of Cardiology*[71] and he would have been so pleased to see it.

The loss of staff took its toll and then the medical school of the University of Zimbabwe was temporarily closed for a year or so in 2008. Never before had it closed since its inception. For the first time in the history of the medical school, the Dean of the Medical school had to approach the South African medical schools to take its final year students. The South African medical schools shared out the 150 students or so but the first to fourth year medical students had to stay at home. I remember a sweet third year medical student called Vimbai, who travelled all the way to Cape Town, some two thousand miles away from Harare, to ask a South African medical school to take her as a third year medical student. A combination of a different medical curriculum and lack of free spaces prevented her from getting a place. The medical school restarted in 2009 and Vimbai proceeded with her studies. I hear that she has since graduated.

---

[71]http://bjcardio.co.uk/2009/01/a-three-dimensional-anatomy-model-of-the-heart-organ-using-a-gloved-hand/

Chapter 16

Trustful Norfolk

I LECTURED ANATOMY FOR AT LEAST the last one and half years while I was in South Africa, and then started my PhD study. The PhD study was a follow up of my Masters work. Six months into my PhD I had to press a "big pause button" to take up a lectureship in anatomy at the University of East Anglia in Norwich, England.

I was offered the post after being short listed. I applied for and was given a work visa from the United Kingdom Embassy in South Africa. One of the lecturers at Medical School in Norwich offered me temporary accommodation while I was organising myself into the new town. The entire relocation took about five months. I had to keep paying in South Africa the rentals for my flat for an extra four months, together with a contract mobile phone for another 14 months. The University of East Anglia fortunately assisted with shipping my personal stuff from South Africa. I swapped my South African licence for a full British driving licence and had a car to use within a month of being in Norwich.

The University of East Anglia was built in 1963 during the time when concrete was very popular. The great bulk of the administration buildings, students' union and academic buildings were built of dull uninspiring and unplastered concrete. My initial impressions of the university were that it looked like some 'communist government buildings'. With time, the concrete has sort of dissolved and I no longer 'see' it. The older student residential buildings were ziggurat-like buildings. Ziggurat buildings were initially made by the Persians and were pyramid shaped terraces and it was usually difficult to work out where the entrance and exit doors were. The architecture at the University of East Anglia has won numerous prizes. Green lawns lie between the ziggurat buildings and a charming lake situated on the campus grounds. I normally take a walk during my lunch times and chit-chat with the fishermen at the lake. The university Sportspark is the largest indoor multi-sports facility in the United Kingdom.

The face of lecturing has matured over the last ten or so years and the technical side of teaching has become more professionalised. A teaching qualification is now required for new lecturers in Britain and is the lecturer's professional equivalent of the teachers' Post Graduate Certificate of Education (PGCE). The PGCE is a compulsory qualification to be a school teacher. Over the last three years, I have applied myself whole-heartedly and passed all the six modules and a research dissertation, entitled *"A preparatory framework for developing a theory on how anatomy is learnt"*. As part of my probation conditions, I had to undertake a compulsory Masters in Higher Education degree (MAHEP). Hopefully with the MAHEP completed, I can re-press the "big pause button" and proceed with my fifth and final degree, a PhD. It is unbelievable that after nine years of studying at university I still have another four years to go! The MAHEP was an eye opener. I was schooled in traditional schools that placed emphasis on teacher-led-teaching in Zimbabwe while the MAHEP is more inclined toward student-led-learning which is usual in the United Kingdom. Having passed the MAHEP, I am now eligible to be a Fellow of the Higher Education Academy of the United Kingdom.

Despite the reputation of Norfolk as a rather insular place today, it has a fascinating history and is today a largely rural county with under 4% non-white residents recorded in the 2001 census. The first notable organised Norfolk residents,[72] from 100 BC, were the native Iceni tribe.[73] Challenged by the Roman Empire, King Prasutagus of the Iceni was defeated in 47 AD, enabling the Romans to rule indirectly until his death in 61 AD. Then, after persecution and harassment, his wife Boudicca (or Boudica), supported by her daughters and tribe, firmly defended the independence of the area. Boudicca boldly led a major uprising that defeated the Roman Ninth Legion, destroyed the capital of Roman Britain in Colchester and razed London to the ground.[74] The Romans had exceptionally advanced technologies ranging from civil construction, military prowess and a highly efficient civil administration. The Romans regrouped within a year or so, conquered the Iceni and ruled until 410 AD.

The Roman Empire eventually became too large to defend and the Anglo-Saxons[75] (comprising of people from Germany, Denmark and northern Holland) held the conquered territory of Norfolk from 410 AD to 1066 AD. The Anglo-Saxons built up the region, including the City of Norwich, only briefly interrupted for 50 years by the Vikings of Scandinavian Denmark, Norway and Sweden from 869 AD.

The French led by King William the Conqueror then took reign over England in the Norman Conquest. The French, for a time, expropriated 95% of the land from the English to French landlords, simultaneously barring the English from holding top positions in government or the church. Norwich Cathedral was

---

[72] http://en.wikipedia.org/wiki/History_of_Norfolk
[73] http://en.wikipedia.org/wiki/Iceni
[74] http://www.bbc.co.uk/history/historic_figures/boudicca.shtml
[75] http://en.wikipedia.org/wiki/History_of_Norfolk#Anglo-Saxon_Norfolk

established early on and is one of the greatest Norman (mediaeval period) buildings in England. Its doorway is marked by a statue to Julian of Norwich,[76] the first woman to write a book in English in 1393, in a period dominated by the French language. Landmarks such as the Norwich Castle (the third castle to be built in the England after the Tower of London and Colchester castle), and the famous Norwich City Walls were built to defend the City. Norwich was the second capital of England for many years thanks largely to its woollen textile trade. The current Queen,[77] Queen Elizabeth II, is the head of the Church of England and the ceremonial Head of State for the United Kingdom and Commonwealth of 16 countries across the world, including Australia and Canada. She is the continuous monarch from the French King William the Conqueror.

Some subtle ways of English towns have taken me a while to perceive. There seems to be a constant theme of trust embedded with a whiff of tradition in everyday life. I have seen some unmanned stalls selling fruit or eggs outside the homes of the sellers, in the villages on the outskirts of Norwich. The stalls tend to have a jar of self-help change for good measure. As far as I have inquired, England must be one of the few nations that allow you to put petrol into your car before you pay money. People from America, continental Europe and Asia were equally surprised at such practices. At the moment, the price of petrol has shot through the roof and is sold for £1.35 per litre, with the taxman unashamedly raking in £0.80 per litre. The high petrol prices have rattled the trust of some people in Norfolk. There have been increased reports of people speeding off without

---

[76]http://en.wikipedia.org/wiki/Julian_of_Norwich
[77]http://www.history-timelines.org.uk/people-timelines/31-timeline-of-english-monarchs.htm
http://www.royal.gov.uk/HMTheQueen/HMTheQueen.aspx

paying for their full tank.[78] I am reminded of a time when I put some petrol into my car and was shaken to find I had forgotten my wallet at home! I went inside the shop and described my predicament to the shop teller. He gave me a slip of paper and asked me to write my name and address on it, without asking for confirmation of my identity, and asked me to come back the following day with the money. He did not check the details I wrote and I could have written anything on it. I came the following day with the money and paid it to a different shop teller. He did not even know that there was someone who had not paid for petrol the previous day!

I am in awe of the number and grandeur of the church buildings in Norwich. Norwich in the 14th century had as many as 60 churches and seven monastic houses wrapped around a wall made of flintstone that had a perimeter of mere two and a half miles. It would take you just over a year if you attended each church on a different Sunday morning.[79] The largest church building is the eleventh-century Anglican Cathedral, although it was initially a Roman Catholic church building for hundreds of years. It was built of flintstone and mortar and was overlaid by cream-coloured Caen limestone. The cathedral is costing a whopping £3700 per day to maintain.[80] The lofty ceilings and the polished organs add to the serenity of the place of worship. The high quality of materials used and the detailed statues, called 'bosses', added to the immense cost of building these churches. The relatively new Roman Catholic Cathedral comes second in terms of size. Building these churches required a lot of sacrifices. There are some reports that some rich landlords invested in the building of cathedrals for the wrong motives, such as prestige and fame. I would expect people who built those churches built

---

[78]http://www.edp24.co.uk/news/norfolk_challenge_to_fuel_theft_1_476943
[79]http://www.norwich-churches.org/Education/education.shtm
[80]http://www.cathedral.org.uk/help/

them out of reverence to God and did not just donate to generate charity mileage among their peers. God examines the heart and not the outward appearance.

The buildings stand as a firm witness of the period and makes Norwich look like a Christian ghost town. As a very crude indication of godliness—or godlessness—in the United Kingdom, I will use church attendance as a measure. A century ago church attendance used to be 70% of the population and the period tallied with the arrival of the first missionaries in Zimbabwe. Robert Moffat, a Scottish man, was the first missionary to work among the Ndebele tribe in the southern part of Zimbabwe between 1845 and 1870. Robert Moffat lived a very frugal life in the tribe lands of Botswana and Zimbabwe and was the most humble person you would ever meet. He was in stark contrast to early colonisers who wanted to line their pockets as quickly as possible, irrespective of whom they had to kill for it. The Robert Tredgold Primary School I attended was named after his great grandson, Robert Clarkson Tredgold.[81] Moffat was the father-in-law to David Livingstone, another famous Scottish explorer rather than missionary. It is also worth mentioning that the Shona word for church is 'kereke' and sounds all too similar to the Scottish word for church, 'kirk'. The similarity most probably arose from the presence of the two Scottish fellows, Robert Moffat and David Livingstone.

I have seen three of the dozen or so statues of David Livingstone. The first is in Victoria Falls in Zimbabwe and is about twice my size. He was the first European to 'discover' the falls and named it after the sitting Queen, Queen Victoria. The second statue is on the Zambian side of Victoria Falls. The third statue I saw of Livingstone is in the Princes Street gardens in Edinburgh in Scotland, close to the main train station. Exploring the source of

---

[81]http://www.dacb.org/stories/southafrica/moffat_johnsmith.html

rivers became David Livingstone's main preoccupation, and his family and missionary work ended up being highly neglected and taking a toll.

The work of the early missionaries is still visible in Zimbabwe. About 90% of the population affiliate themselves with Christianity. Mission hospitals provide free treatment to about 10% of sick patients and mission boarding schools form about 30% of all the boarding schools in Zimbabwe. The Christians in Norwich, a century or two ago would turn in their graves if they realised that less than 5% of Norwich people ever attend church. Some of the very churches they toiled so hard to build now have nothing to do with God. Indeed, some old church buildings have been given over to nightclubs, karate clubs[82], puppet theatres![83], and another one is being earmarked for clowns[84], despite numerous churches looking for permanent premises in Norwich and are using schools, community and commercial halls.[85]

The hearts of young people seeking for God have been falling, especially in the outskirts of Norwich. Christianity is struggling to resonate with the young. God is now regarded as the God of the aged and is felt to be more relevant to the older rural congregations of Norfolk, with the average age of people attending church, currently 61 years, while the percentage of the population attending church has dropped from 10% to 5% over a thirty-year period. Poland and Ireland still have church attendances of about 70% of the population.[86] The lack of young

[82]http://www.nama4kicks.co.uk/index.html
[83]http://www.puppettheatre.co.uk/about-us
[84]http://www.eveningnews24.co.uk/news/plans_to_turn_empty_norwich_church_st_l aurence_into_a_circus_1_1175148
[85] Such as Norwich Family Life Church, English Reformed Church, Redeemed Christian Church of God, Proclaimers Norwich Church, Servants Church, Norwich Vineyard, Living Waters Pentecostal Fellowship and Queens Community Church.
[86]http://www.whychurch.org.uk/trends.php

people in congregations makes it hard for a young person to join that church as they feel they will not 'connect' with people who are not at the same life stage. The training conduits for young vicars or pastors are equally drying up and it is a spiritual time bomb which is not helping matters. If the current elderly are to pass away, rural Norfolk will enter an unprecedented spiritual era, perhaps in twenty odd years or so.

I am reminded of my time in Zimbabwe, where churches are mainly filled with young people, especially in the cities. I was on record for saying that I spent an average of four months before noticing anyone with significant white hair. Perhaps of the hundred odd pastors in Zimbabwe I have ever heard preaching, only three or so were actually aged above 50 years. The majority of pastors were in their twenties and thirties and burning with a passion for God. This made it easy for them to be relevant to the youth. My experiences and observations in South Africa were similar to the Zimbabwean setting.

Perhaps the religious mumbo-jumbo 'preached' so often today has not been made clear enough. We have all fallen short of the very nature and glory of God. At best, our efforts to be and stay righteous before God, are as filthy rags before God. There are men and women who have represented God and who have stumbled due to temptation, but that does not nullify God. If someone drops out of university, that does not mean the university is bogus. Things such as being environmentally friendly, keeping fit, doing charitable work, attending church services and donating to worthy causes do not garner any righteousness with God. God has set aside one door for us to be righteous with Him. He sacrificed His Son Jesus to take the sins of all of us. Jesus has been made the sole and only way to achieve righteousness with God. God currently speaks very clearly to 'each and every person' he has a relationship with through His Holy Spirit. The relationship will lead you to be at peace with God and not leave you with a horrible conscience gnawing at you because of sin. The sense of purpose of your life as to why you were created will grow clearer. The pursuit of worldly targets will not remove the sense of pointlessness and absurdity, for we are eternal beings and we all know that nothing will stub out that knowledge. At times when men have pleased God, He has done miracles. The prophesies God made in the past have not ever failed. The future Bible prophesies and new prophesies that are being spoken of in our age will come to pass. There will be a day of reckoning. These are matters on my heart.

In all my travels, I am yet to see a more charitable people than the people living in Norfolk. Without fail, weekly collections of clothing that people no longer need are collected on my street. Occasionally some young lads knock on my doors requesting monthly donations of a few pounds monthly to charities, such as 'Cancer research', children's and animal charities. Even the Government encourages donations to charities by topping the donation by an extra 28% of donations by tax payers. There are dozens of shops in Norwich, which sell clothing, furniture, and other household items in good condition. Men and women who take exceptional pride in volunteering their time to work for the charity shops man the shops. Sadly such charitable movements across the country are unheard of in Zimbabwe and South Africa.

Roads are never pretty straightforward in Norfolk. There are a few single straight roads, probably less than five roads out of the thousands of roads in Norfolk. The most conspicuous token straight road is a stretch of road of a couple of miles connecting the town of Acle to Great Yarmouth. Each and every other road warps a little to the right and then swings back to the left, if at all it returns. What lies ahead of the twists and turns is further made more hazardous by the glaring absence of space on the edges of the road. Cars literally get a massage from the shrubs on the edge of the road when driving along. The heavy presence of roundabouts does not help the linearity of the roads and have been used to replace traffic lights, although some of the roundabouts are heavily sprinkled with traffic lights nonetheless. The non-linear roads make my perceptions of directions an uphill task. Oh, how I miss the grid road system of perpendicular roads of Bulawayo!

There are three places in Norfolk that make my heart all warm and fuzzy. The first is a quiet and solitary picnic bench in Bawburgh village, some two miles west of the University of East Anglia. The bench is on the greenest lawn in Norfolk and has the sound of a river stream trickling a few yards away to soothe the nerves. Big trees provide leafy shade and there is a traffic sign with a duck to warn drivers to be careful of harming the ducks around the picnic place. On the other side of the stream is a pasture for sheep. Oh, what a good spot to be at peace with yourself, far away from the rat race I lead in Norwich.

My second favourite tourist place is a day boat hire on the Norfolk broads, a network of rivers of over a hundred navigable miles. The Broads were once filled with peat. The peat was an accumulation of partially decayed grass and other vegetation that was dug up and used as fuel. The peat excavations left were then flooded up creating the Norfolk Broads. The owners of boats are always trustful that the public will return the boats safely. It is an amazing excursion through the Norfolk countryside on that picnic boat.

The third place I rate very highly is the area made up by both the Upper and Lower Sheringham towns. Upper Sheringham Gardens are gorgeous in April when the selected rhododendrons, a collection of shrubs and small trees that flower in full bloom, produce a Disney garden feel. The walk along the beach of the Lower Sheringham town is one of the most tranquil in Norfolk.

I have had my fair share of touring around Britain, from the quiet Belfast in Northern Ireland, modern looking Cardiff in Wales, gothic buildings in Edinburgh and the once mighty industrial powerhouse, Glasgow in Scotland. Various places in England, such as Sheffield, Suffolk, London and the university towns of Oxford and Cambridge, have made an impression on me. Of all the places in Britain, I would rate highly the west coast of Scotland, where a Scottish friend invited me. My mother, who was visiting England for four months from Zimbabwe at the time of the invite, was excited to go and her excitement grew as we made our way there. The family of my friend owned a Bed and Breakfast lodge in Carradale.[87] We travelled by train from Norwich to Edinburgh and along the way my mother saw the sea for the first time in her life, the North Sea. She greatly feared that the houses near the sea would be flooded. I calmed her fears by saying, "These houses have been there for hundreds of years."

We spent two days sightseeing in places in Edinburgh and Glasgow, such as the Scottish Parliament and Edinburgh Castle. A four-hour drive from Glasgow to Carradale, after a brief rest in Claclan, snaked around numerous lakes and steep mountains to reach the west coast of Scotland. We were so west of Scotland that we could see the northern coastline of Northern Ireland. The village of Carradale was so small that the only bank there, the Royal Bank of Scotland, only opened for one hour on Thursdays at 11a.m. Carradale village has a small harbour, plenty of mountain hikes with breath-taking views and was within easy reach of the islands of Arran and Gigha.[88] We spent a day cycling the length of Gigha and exploring the acclaimed Gigha Gardens. Gigha island is a mere seven miles long and three miles wide

---

[87]http://www.refreshingscotland.co.uk/page4.htm

[88]Gigha (pronounced Giya) means 'God's Island' in Gaelic, a Scottish traditional language.

with beautiful white sandy beaches. On another day, we completed a local hike that provided us with stunning views of the Island of Arran and the coastline of Northern Ireland, while I was wearing my traditional African Lesotho hat! For my mother, this trip was a highlight of her time spent in the United Kingdom. I hope to be able to return soon to such tranquil, untamed and sparsely populated lands such as western Scotland.

Chapter 17

The Worth of the Human Body

I HAVE SEEN SOME OF THE GLORIOUS and astonishing attributes of the human body, in my time as an anatomist and physiotherapist, that are of such beauty and complexity that words cannot fully portray. The body is run by smart programmes that each in turn are monitored and controlled by other clever programmes. The source of the programmes is a two-metre long string of genetic material, called DNA for short, that is tightly super coiled into a minuscule cell. If you look very carefully at your fingerprint lines on your finger, each width of the lines is loaded with about fifty cells across. Each DNA strand is only made up of four letters or tools that are randomly repeated until the chain has billions of letters. The set-up is perfected art!

I find it a complete marvel that the four simple letters are able to design a baby's face that is similar to that of her dad. Just imagine building a skyscraper with only four things, e.g. a spade, a brick, glass and glue, to such an extent that the skyscraper will be able to move, heal itself and reproduce smaller buildings after nine months of 'pregnancy'. A true wonder indeed! There are three things of the human body derived from these four tools that stand out the most from all the other things made by DNA; namely, the address directory that governs where each should be located, the emotional photocopying headquarters, and the clocks all over our bodies. There are tens of trillions of cells in a body and they all seem to know their home address where they should be located. If they all crowded in a popular spot, then that area will have a tumour and that will be undesirable. Each and every molecule and atom in the body is completely replaced every seven years because of normal wear and tear. The process is carried out so diligently and meticulously that the addresses of the cells are not shuffled or jumbled up, otherwise you would not recognise the face of a friend you last saw seven years ago. Chopping off some of the cells, as happens when getting a bruise, is not enough to confuse the cell address system and the healed skin becomes identical to the undamaged skin. The complexity and tranquillity of the cells is mind blowing. As mankind, we still do not know much about the cell despite having made huge scientific strides.

There is an emotional photocopying centre of operations (headquarters, if you like) in the brain, formally called the limbic system, that controls emotion. What amazes me is how the four tools can program the emotional photocopying headquarters to photocopy 100% of the emotions in another person. If you happen to see someone who was robbed ten minutes ago, you will feel 100% of what he is feeling. The next time you attend a wedding, try to temporarily look at the faces of the rest of the church while the groom is kissing the bride to see the extent of emotional photocopying among the congregation. Seasoned beggars are very skilled in hijacking the emotional photocopying and make you photocopy their difficult situation. A seasoned actor can easily captivate the audience and infectiously spread the sadness or humour of a play.

The four tools go on to make clocks of every kind that lie in the body. The clocks trigger puberty at around ten to twelve years of age in most of us and white hair starts popping up when people reach their thirties. It is no wonder that most of us spend nine months in pregnancy because of these clocks. Some clocks only monitor hours and minutes. If someone asked you how long you have been cooking, or talking, you can give a realistic answer of let us say 20 minutes because of these very clocks that run in the background. Some clocks even monitor seconds. Top classical musicians will detect a misplaced musical note instantly if it is played a fraction of a second too early or too late.

It is when I am in the throes of being cognisant of these three marvels that my stomach turns and becomes unsettled due to some undertakings that are secretly done in the United Kingdom in general. The relatively casual approach to, and the large scale of abortions in the United Kingdom has knocked me sideways, like a massive cultural shock of the highest order. The United Kingdom has one of the most lenient and liberal laws for abortion.[89] Any reason given to the doctor is valid enough to initiate the abortion operation in the National Health Service and can be carried out within the first twenty weeks of pregnancy, whereas most counties in Europe limit it to twelve weeks. Reasons such as being unemployed or that looking after a baby will be a mental burden are good enough reasons. Consequently the United Kingdom has one of the highest abortion rates in the whole world despite being the most supportive country in the world to assist single mothers financially. Single mothers in the United Kingdom are almost guaranteed free council housing, child tax credits and other assistance. It simply does not add up!

The total abortion rates for the United Kingdom are a whopping 200 000 per year against a number of 700 000 actually born every year. Just to convey a better grasp of the numbers, let us assume that if an average sized primary school has an annual intake of one hundred grade one pupils every year, then 2000 primary schools will be needed across the country to school the number of unborn babies killed off. The number of foetuses with severe abnormalities are generally less than 2000 per year. It is now a fact that one in every three women in the United Kingdom

---

[89]http://www.bpas.org/bpaswoman/abortion

over the age of forty-five has had an abortion.[90] The burden is on all of us really. Some spineless men become insensible to their sweethearts on hearing that they are a few weeks pregnant and desert them. The communities we live in need to be as supportive of babies and children, while line managers will need to be a little bit more lenient and understanding of the demands mothers and fathers face. Notwithstanding what everyone else should be doing, it is important to be cognisant of the fact that the mother and father should pull their weight and know that the onus of raising up the child rests squarely on both of them.

An abortion very sadly shuts down the address directory that governs where each cell should be located, switches off all the various clocks in the body and dissembles the emotional photocopy machine. A very sad day indeed! I have heard of the loss of humans on an even larger scale.

I was taught my O-level History by a Welsh lady, Ms Evans, and learned of World Affairs since 1919 to the Cold War. It covered the aftermath of World War One, such as the Treaty of Versailles, to before and after World War Two, and to the 'Ho Chi Minh trail' of the Vietnam War. History has helped me understand some of the underlying social currents and dynamics of modern-day Europe and the world. So I knew that Eastern Europe was kind of different from Western Europe and so I chose to tour Belgium and Poland in April of 2010. I chose Belgium because it had the most efficient Schengen visa processing department among the group of Schengen countries and I felt it would give me a glimpse of Western Europe. It took the embassy in London two days to process a visa application, but as I learnt while on the ropes, that African passports are further posted to Belgium and the process took three weeks

---

[90] http://www.dailymail.co.uk/news/article-82368/Third-women-abortion-age-45.html

instead! I impatiently waited for the visa. It duly arrived and I was ready to set off.

I took the Eurostar train to Brussels city, which was elegantly set up, and looked imposing. The presence of the European Parliament and the strong euro, which was electively trading on par with the British pound, made Brussels very pricey. Brussels is best toured on one of the day long cycle tours. The behemoth and massive Brussels Palace of Justice building, the size of three football pitches, was the largest 19th century building in Europe.[91] A black bronze sculpture copy of the 'Manneken Pis', an overrated foot-tall statue of a young boy with previous versions having been stolen over hundreds of years, and the European Parliament are the main tourist nuggets of Brussels. In addition, I visited what is probably the finest looking town square in Europe, the Grand Place, and indulged in some of the rightly rated fresh, moist Belgium chocolates. The next city was Brugge and I can confidently say that Brugge town is the most charming and romantic town I have ever seen. I would not go there alone again. Virtually all the houses in the main part of the city are over a hundred or two hundred years old and the town sits on a network of manmade rivers, graced with boats loaded with camera-happy tourists whizzing through it. The last Belgian city I visited was Antwerp, the diamond capital of the world. Much to my surprise I was told that seventy percent of the diamonds in the world are traded in the city. I had thought the South African company De Beers was the maestro of the diamond world. I proceeded with my tour to Poland.

The main place I wanted to see in Poland was the Auschwitz Concentration Camp and the nearest city to it is Krakow, Poland's second biggest city. Krakow was the oldest capital city of a once much larger and powerful Poland. Accommodation and

[91] http://en.wikipedia.org/wiki/Law_Courts_of_Brussels

restaurant prices were a full third of England's prices and most of the young hotel staff spoke English. An eight-hundred-year-old salt mine, Wieliczka Salt Mine, is a UNESCO World Heritage Site, graced with over two hundred miles of tunnels and even has a salt Cathedral in part of the mine. In the heydays of the salt mine, salt was worth more than gold—which explains the myriad of extensive tunnels.

Nothing could have ever prepared me for the grinding human desperation that was apparent at the Auschwitz Concentration camp I toured, another UNESCO World Heritage Site. The camp had eighty wooden cabins that were each twenty-five feet wide by one hundred feet long. The cabins were designed for basic bunker beds to house one hundred people but had one thousand people cramped in each of them at the height of the Second World War, without the luxury of heating or a toilet. The whole camp had about 80 000 prisoners in an area of four football stadiums. The newly built Wembley Football Stadium in London holds 90 000 spectators during star-studded games.

There were three groups of prisoners, those in the wooden cabins, those who came by train and the Sonderkommandos prisoners. The food was intentionally made so subhuman that it was common for the prisoners to be given bread slices made from flour mixed with wood shavings to make the intestines bleed and get infected. The luxury of using an open public toilet was granted for ten minutes at 7a.m. each morning and a nature call at any other time elicited a bullet from the guards and the average survival rate was three months. Different colour badge codes added to the hopelessness and humiliation. The prisoners were classified as Jew (the largest group), homosexuals, Blacks and political prisoners.

The second group of prisoners were brought in by trains from all over Europe to be exterminated. They were tricked into taking a shower after a gruelling two or four day train ride without any rest to stretch themselves, were gassed in the shower rooms and cremated to destroy the evidence. Probably four to six million persons were gassed and cremated into thin air, with very little physical trace of them remaining, save for the meticulous documents of the Nazi that survived from being destroyed in the closing days of the war.

The last group of prisoners were the Sonderkommandos prisoners. Their daily chores were intolerable, and how they met their end is too horrifying to convey graphically for the readers of this book and is the worst thing anyone could imagine. The camp was designed by Nazi Germans for people they considered far below animals in worth, that we reconsidered responsible for all the ills of the country. Perhaps this has taught us the dangers of self-importance of a particular people over others. The reasons for the passivity and callousness of the generality of the German civic society to suffering groups still need to be nicely explained to me. The German guards who guarded these prisoners went home every evening to their families and had normal middle class lives.

Chapter 18

The 'Fattened Lions'
Restricting Education

N EVER BEFORE IN MY LIFE have I ever visualised the
'fattened lions' so clearly as now. The fattened lions almost
exclusively hunt children who are brought up in family
backgrounds without professional adults. There are seven
fattened lions prowling and seeking whom they may devour.

The first lion, the 'victim lion', is the noisiest and probably, the
easiest to spot and to locate in the educational jungle. The lion
roams without any purpose and is always in a bad mood because
some unknown creature traumatised it when it was still a chubby
cub. The 'trauma' affected its ability to hunt. Now, as a grown up
lion, it is among the thinnest of lions. When it looks at the rest of
the lion clan, all the other lions seem to have fluffier fur and
rounder eyes than itself. The soul of the 'victim lion' sinks a little
when it sees patches of its fur falling off and its thin hide
exposing the sticking out ribs. "Someone just has to pay!" roars
the vicious lion. He becomes so preoccupied with getting his
revenge that he no longer goes with the clan during the late
afternoon hunts but remains roaming aimlessly the rest of the
day.

Had I been torn apart by the 'victim lion', I might very easily
have taken the golden opportunity of writing the current book to
'name and shame' all the people on both sides of the

Mediterranean Sea who made my life go through rough patches. But I have refrained from this because I have escaped the 'victim lion'.

The second fattened lion, the 'prejudicial lion', has the sharpest pair of eyes capable of telling apart even very subtle colours. The lion can tell apart the more yellowish deer from the more brownish deer. It has a larger appetite for the more yellowish deer. Somehow, somehow the 'prejudicial lion' can see the colour of the fur of the deer from a good mile away even on a misty day. The 'prejudicial lion' is the most efficient lion and no single deer with a yellowish tinge has ever escaped alive after being seen.

Some societal institutions have placed glass ceilings that reduce social mobility, and the glass ceilings are the 'prejudicial lions'. The 'prejudicial lions' have ensured that those youths from non-professional families feel uncomfortable with some aspects of lifestyles in higher educational training institutions and may feel embarrassed to seek for advice and mentorship help concerning the social issues that are affecting their ability to focus on their school or university work. Looking for a job, while having no professional contacts or advice, can be a challenge and they have lower chances of landing a professional internship or summer job. While attending a job interview, a broad accent or too many scars on your face might act as the yellowish tinge as part of your fur and will attract the wrath of the 'prejudicial lions.'

A notable example of 'prejudicial lion' behaviour arises from my experiences with the Prestige Barclays Bank in Zimbabwe. I remember so very vividly the time I was working as a Physiotherapist and a Junior Anatomy lecturer in Harare, Zimbabwe. I had been running a normal bank account for about half a decade with Barclays Bank, ever since I was a first-year student at university. I then accidentally came across the knowledge that there was a parallel Barclays banking universe called Prestige Current account banking.[92] The account appeared too good to be true, and so I made a half-hearted application. They checked my references and phoned me to let me know that I was given the nod to join. 'Prestige Banking' had its exclusive separate queue-less banking offices. It had comfy sofas to rest your soul, and orange juice or tea to sooth your throat. No proof of identity, such as identity documents or passports, was required, as we were personally known. If there was something wrong with the account or there was a bounced cheque, they gave me a personal call to my mobile phone. Now that is what I call banking service! If just anyone entered the Prestige Banking offices to open an account, he or she would be taken round in circles until he or she gave up joining.

Towards the middle of 2004, I ran into a financial emergency after securing a job interview for a Lectureship in Anatomy at the University of East Anglia in Norwich and had seven days to be in Norwich from Zimbabwe. I rocked up at the Prestige Banking offices and verbally asked for a pile of cold cash for the flight. The following day they gave me a 'loan' and I flew and stayed a week in the United Kingdom and came back. I only got to complete the loan paperwork after I came back, and repaid the loan in full on my next payday. On that occasion I was a deer with a yellowish tinge that had miraculously been missed by the banking system, which was the 'prejudicial fattened lion'.

The third 'uncharted lion' is very hard to describe because no deer has ever seen it. It lives in the part of the educational jungle that was discovered the last and is called the 'uncharted territory'. No maps exist and it is unsearchable even on a Google-map. The hunting success rates of the 'lions of the uncharted territory' are legendary and the escape rates of the deer

---

[92]http://www.barclays.com/africa/zimbabwe/prestige.htm

are said to be very slim. A good example of battling against the 'uncharted lions' comes from the sandwich filling generation.

I have become extremely proud of the 'sandwich filling generation' of Black Zimbabweans who were born between 1970 and 1985. They were the first mass generation to study A-levels and take up higher education like university degrees. Imagine a sandwich made up of three parts: a bottom bread slice, a sandwich filling and a top bread slice. The bottom bread slice represents the generation of Black A-level pupils, born prior to 1970 before the 'sandwich filling generation' who attended two schools in Zimbabwe (Fletcher High and Goromonzi High School). These two schools were the only schools in the whole country that was allowed by the colonial government to educate Blacks up to A-level, and had an annual intake of eighty odd students. The number of A-level places shot up to over ten thousand a few years after Independence and became the 'sandwich filling generation'.

The unpredicted economic decline at the end of the millennium became the top bread slice to close off the sandwich filling generation. Those of the sandwich filling generation gave a good account of themselves against the 'fattened lions' of the educational territory, despite having no older persons as mentors or setting the precedence. Over 50% of my O-level classmates at Milton High have completed technical or university level education. Two of my former classmates have finished PhDs while four of them are ploughing through their PhD studies. About 70% of my A-level stream at Fletcher High School went to universities in Zimbabwe the year after getting their A-level results. I have narrated my experiences in the world of anatomy and physiotherapy in the earlier chapters and show how much we were among the first generation to graduate. I have made online searches of all my university lecturers at the University of Zimbabwe and they have hardly published abroad. My scientific manuscript submitted to British and American medical journals was indeed a big step into the 'uncharted territory'.

I have been warned about 'uncharted lions' that lurk in England. England is one of the most difficult countries to achieve a Professorship as a Black person. I have asked over 40 of my Norwich friends and mates if they have ever seen or heard of a Black Professor in real life or even in a TV documentary. They said they have never seen one. I then made a major search on the internet and only managed to find one Black professor, who was not even British born, but a Malawian.[93] After a long search, a work colleague led me to a news article on a website that said there are only 50 Black Professors out of 14 400 lecturers in Britain. Somewhere along the professional path there are exceptional sloppy paths that virtually all do not manage to go beyond.

The fourth fattened lion, the 'translucent lion', is the most powerful and extremely difficult to spot. Behold it is completely translucent and has an unrestricted access to deer on the educational savannah. Virtually all the deer have the tell-tale scars of being pounced upon by the 'translucent lion'. The translucent lions literally sleep and move with the deer herd and have ensured that they are among the fattest lions in the land. The 'translucent lion' represents the unconscious damping effect that the parents or local surroundings have imparted to their children over an eighteen-year period that starts from birth. These deer represent some of the lads that would have failed to get their dream birthday presents or those single parents that cannot afford groceries beyond the generic plain vanilla, Tesco and Asda products. Hobbies after school activities and sports gear are heavily pruned to the bare activities that can proceed with just sunshine and playmates. Tantrums are frequent in early years

---

[93] http://www.southampton.ac.uk/socsci/about/staff/njm2.page

until the children are old enough to realise the financial pain they are causing to the parents, if the tantrums are to be heeded. In time, the choice of food, clothing, hobbies and even the type of career training become permanently depressed to a basic and easiest level.

My neighbourhood of Mzilikazi, where I spent my childhood, was a massive destroyer of career aspirations. Of my generation of children from the neighbourhood of some two hundred children, only three managed to go to university. The son of Magistrate Mapani, my older brother Bryan and I were the only three who went to university. Had Bryan not gone to university, I doubt that I would have gone. He is now a water engineer in Darwin, Australia. People do not readily appreciate the influence family members and the community have on you. We tend to pick up on usual things surrounding us simply because everyone is doing it. We all like to feel part of the group and copy each other. Although I was sad to have left Mzilikazi, looking back in hindsight I find that moving out of that neighbourhood upgraded my job mentality from that of earning monthly wages to that of making a difference through a professional career in a tremendous way.

The 'expect-the-least-out-of-you lion' can greatly discourage a pupil. A schoolteacher may behave as an 'expect-the-least-out-you lion' by labelling a pupil as 'hopeless' or saying 'it runs in the family', and that can haunt a pupil for life. The 'expect-the-least-out-you lion' sees deer as a much inferior and lowly creature who should not aspire to anything beyond the grass of the jungle. It believes the deer should settle for the leftovers of society. The last priorities for everyone else are assumed to be good enough as the first choice for the deer. Words addressed to us either build us or tear us apart. A collective reinforcement to take the leftovers of the choices has a strong tendency for us to live up to those words.

The least desirable career choices tend to be monotonous and boring. Choosing careers you are passionate about and can do well in is more likely to be fun to do and offer you better chances of excelling in that field.

Avoid the danger of choosing a career for money because after you have bought the materialistic things you have craved for, let us say after a year or two, what will motivate you to wake up at six o'clock sharp in the dead of winter to go to work?

The 'we-and-them' fattened lions highlight the social categorisation and social class problems we impose on ourselves. The 'we-and-them' lion is best illustrated by the 'Norfolk fence'. The 'Norfolk fence' exists in the very heart of Norfolk and is an average looking real fence that separates aspirations in a massive way. It is a two metre-high fence and is about half a mile long. The Sportspark end of the fence is the most visible part while a thicket of trees obscures the fence at the other end. There is no gap or gate to allow people or aspirations to cross over. On one side of the fence lies the best university in the Norfolk country, the University of East Anglia which is listed among the 200 top universities in the world. On the other side of the 'Norfolk fence' lies Earlham High School. The school has literary one of the least desirable O-level and A-level results in the whole of the Norfolk country. A mere 14% of the pupils were getting five O-levels and about 40% of the pupils had special educational needs.[94] The results are not acceptable.

[94]http://news.bbc.co.uk/1/shared/bsp/hi/education/06/school_tables/secondary_schools/html/926_gcse_lea.stm and http://news.bbc.co.uk/1/shared/bsp/hi/education/06/school_tables/secondary_schools/html/926_4068.stmandhttp://www.norwich.gov.uk/intranet_docs/corporate/public/committee/reports/2009/Scrutiny/REP_Scrutiny_Earlham_High_School_Consultation_2009_02_12.pdf

There is hope. The results were so bad that the Norfolk County Council decided to rebrand the Earlham High School and be formally called the City Academy Norwich. The City Academy Norwich received a shot in the arm of £21 million in December 2010.[95] When I am passing through the school I see the construction of new buildings in full swing. Things are looking up and last year's results (2011 year) produced an O-level pass rate of 40%, despite the school having pupil catchment areas that are among some of the most socially deprived (across seven factors[96]) residential areas in Norfolk county.[97] Key feeder primary schools to the City Academy Norwich, such as Bluebell Primary School, are among the weakest academic primary schools in Norfolk.[98] It will take the principal Mr David Brunton and his staff some years to tilt the balance. A single year will not rectify the deficits of many years.

I really wonder at the contrast between pupils having low aspirations and university students with high career aspirations. The catchment area of the school is actually the residential area closest to the university where most students live. Thus the pupils of the school live in the same residential area as the students that go to the University of East Anglia. The school pupils and the university students use the same city council services, use the same hospital and buy from the same shops—yet the career aspirations are worlds apart.

The difference in aspiration may be that the pupils are seeing themselves though the 'we-and-them' glasses. The 'we-and-

[95] http://www.bbc.co.uk/news/uk-england-norfolk-12057829
[96] Income, employment, health and disability, education, skills and training, barriers to housing and services, living environment and crime
[97] http://norfolkinsight.org.uk/dataviews/report?reportId=80&viewId=120&geoRepor tId=2494&geoId=12&geoSubsetId=
[98] http://www.bbc.co.uk/news/special/education/school_tables/primary/11/html/eng_maths_926.stm?compare=

them' fattened lions mauled me a lot during my primary and secondary days. I hope you detected the 'we-and-them' theme from my earlier primary and secondary school chapters. I felt part of 'them' from high school onwards. I honestly think that a programme that is meant to raise the aspirations in education should make the pupils and the organisers feel they are on the same social side. The more we have people from the same community pushing programmes for career aspirations, rather than parachuting one-day programmes from outside the cultural and social terrain, the better we will stop the 'we-and-them lions'. It is so important for the organisers to dress more casually to make the student or pupil 'participants' feel at home, rather than wearing very formal clothing that might suggest a social or cultural dichotomy. I also think that it is important for the pupils to have a 'them' mentality and that may help in raising aspirations.

The seventh lion is the 'unskilled work lion'. I have noticed a very aggressive tendency of people from non-professional families to remain in unskilled work that does not require any training. I would cordially encourage anyone to take up a career as a professional tradesmen, such as being a plumber or electrician. I feel that the public and policy makers in the United Kingdom have under-rated these professionals. It takes many years of training and apprenticeship for someone to swiftly trouble shoot an electrical fault in a house or a car refusing to start. These tradespersons are now commanding fees that make physicians and solicitors turn green with envy—given that the minimum wage in the United Kingdom for anyone working a full eight-hour day shift is about £50. I have had a number of pleasant experiences with tradesmen while in Norwich. A socket in my bedroom developed a fault some time ago and the electrician I called out pocketed £70 for a fifteen-minute job. The cheapest non-dealer mechanic I could find for my troublesome Vauxhall Omega car was £40 per hour. The car has bled me dry and I have spent over £3000 in all sorts of repairs on it over the last two years. The best bargain price I could find for a gas annual inspection certificate for inspecting my gas stove in a snappy ten minutes was £68.

I grew up in a country where everything was repaired, whether it was a watch or fridge with a fault, or a torn shoe. Each and every home had a needle and thread for stitching together a torn shirt. The main motive was to reduce unnecessary costs and such a strategy would probably not work in England today because of the relatively high wages, even if the skills became available. However, paradoxically, instead of encouraging the spirit of repairing, there is a great drive to reduce our carbon print and recycle things. The rainbow colours of the plethora of city council bins on the streets on a waste collection day testify to this. I feel there is a niche role for tradesmen skilled in repairing products to hide behind the spirit of reducing carbon footprints in England.

Chapter 19

Reflections on My Own Education

THE BENEFITS OF EDUCATION take a long, long time to achieve. It is very unfortunate that some extremely short-sighted people will not commit themselves to training or a certificate because there is no short-term reward. These people think that the fruits of education are a mighty castle in the air and so settle to become a stick in the mud. Maybe you are in your secondary school and wondering what the point is of the long hours of homework that is as dull as dishwater and is due tomorrow. It is only now that I can fully appreciate the full impact of having a decent and solid education during my secondary schooling. The English I learnt taught me to write joined up sentences and realise when to use the appropriate words from among words that sound similar like 'whose/who's', 'later/latter' and 'phantom/fathom'. I doubt if I would have had the courage to write a public book like this one in my fifth language, English. Back then I thought English Literature was an absolute waste of time and was overrated. The concepts of English Literature are now proving handy and has lent colour to this current book. My love for mathematics paid off. The importance of the mathematics I learnt enabled me to survive for three years on money I made from teaching private mathematics lessons. I had nothing to learn in my A-level Mathematics during my first year because of the labours I had put into my O-level Additional Mathematics.

The history I learnt opened my eyes to the things that occurred in the past and helped me to place the relevant history at various intervals of this current book. Geography has contributed immensely into me getting more from my holiday travels across the world later on in life, from massive limestone caves in Outdshoorn in South Africa to the Rift Valleys in Eastern Africa. Geography awakened my passion for UNESCO World Heritage Sites, some of which I have visited. The sites are a good tourist place to start when visiting different countries. The different science subjects I have so much loved lay the solid foundations for my career in science. I have used the French I learnt in my travels to various French speaking countries and to talk to French speakers I have met in English-speaking countries. Although I was terrible in written Ndebele, my understanding of Ndebele helped me understand when any Nguni people were speaking, like the Xhosas in Cape Town, the Zulus in South Africa, the Swazis in Swaziland and the Ngoni in Malawi. While I did not enjoy all the subjects, I managed to plough in a decent hour's work whenever I was required to.

I normally studied my books and did my homework during primary and secondary schooling while sitting in front of a noisy television, for there was no study room among the various relatives I grew up with. I only had a quiet study desk when I was in boarding at high school, but it was too late—I had become accustomed to reading in noisy environments and to this very day I cannot do any serious studying without earphones on or something.

Truancy is a bad idea. In all my primary and secondary schooldays I was absent from school for no more than five days. I was once absent from school for a week because I had come down with infectious measles and my body was itching. I do not remember any of my parents coming to a school's Parent

Consultation Day but that did not blunt my keenness for education.

Education changes the profile of your circle of friends in a massive way. I have had a look at the names of the people in the phone book of my mobile phone. It has over 600 names. About 70 of the 100 people from Zimbabwe are university graduates, including my relatives. A similar proportion is found among my friends from South Africa and 200 of the 250 are graduates. Less that 10% of all the people I am acquainted with in Norwich do not have a degree. It is not that I have been actively screening out non-graduates but it is something I am becoming aware of as I write this book. There are a few people who combine two professions like myself. Being a Physiotherapist has generated lots of acquaintances and friends in the physiotherapy and occupational therapy fields. I still remember explaining in simple terms what physiotherapy was and was not, repeatedly to different relatives and friends when I initially chose the physiotherapy degree. However, being an anatomist has generated the most of my graduate friends. I taught four generations of health graduates at the medical school of the University of Zimbabwe and three generations of health graduates at the University of Cape Town. I have now spent three years teaching medical, physiotherapy and occupational therapy students at the University of East Anglia. My heavy involvement with church activities involving students at the three universities has also greatly increased my number of graduate friends.

Most of my friends have noticed I do not mention any work or professional inclinations in social circles, for I do not wish to make people unnecessarily conscious of educational background. Being in such an environment of professional people, I find it so much easier to get free professional advice from my mates on legal, architectural, medical or computer matters. I just send them a Facebook message and the answer is sent by the end of the day.

I did not foresee all these changes when I was writing my school homework in primary and secondary school. I only saw a university student for the first time when I was in secondary school because basically none of the older generation had gone to university. And so this has been a big jump!

Education is not everything. It is simply a key that allows you access to particular jobs. Too many people expect miracles from someone who has attended school or has a certain qualification. Nowhere in the educational chain is anyone taught how to be a good parent and yet there is an expectation that professional parents make better parents. Neither is morality taught to everyone who pursues O-levels. To be fair, probably everyone who is in prison passed through the schooling system. Many reasons have been given for the causes of the embarrassing lootings and arsons in England during 2011. The disturbances started after a Black youth, Mark Duggan, was shot dead in Tottenham (London) by the police, and the mayhem spread not only to multiple places in London, but also major cities in England. The reasons given for the mayhem range from lack of youth programmes, the absence of police, poor race relations, welfare dependence, absent fathers, unemployment, gang culture, social irresponsibility, the underclass and downright criminal behaviour.

I personally think that the disturbances all boil down to a "slow-motion moral collapse" and constitute a wakeup call to all of us.[99] The looters have laid a high moral standard for all of us. How many of us will stop unjustly enriching ourselves, in a position of need, when we can literally get away with it? How many of us will return the excess change from a shop teller or avoid reporting for work with a headache, knowing very well that

---

[99]http://www.telegraph.co.uk/news/uknews/crime/8701371/UK-riots-David-Cameron-confronts-Britains-moral-collapse.html

no physician can detect a headache on an X-ray or hospital test? How many of us will not break the speed limit knowing very well that there is no speed camera on a particular stretch of road? The answers to these questions are not found in our general education and will come from our honesty and conscience.

Perhaps there are fewer more fortunate people in the world who got off very lightly than myself in terms of student loans. I had a total student loan debt of $Zim160 000 when I graduated from the University of Zimbabwe in 2003 with the BSc Honours Physiotherapy and BSc Intercalated Honours Human Anatomy degrees. I fully paid off the student loan debt of $Zim160 000 three months after graduating with a bank cheque. The student loans were interest free and the high inflation had tremendously boosted the salaries and made paying back the loans easier. By then a new shirt was $Zim80 000 and hence I paid with a new shirt each of my BSc Honours Physiotherapy and BSc Intercalated Honours Human Anatomy degrees, which were of world class standard. The physiotherapy degree enabled me to register on the United Kingdom Health Professions Council as a Physiotherapist without needing examinations and the anatomy degree paved the way for my career in anatomy at the University of East Anglia. I self-funded myself for the Masters in Medicine in Anatomy degree and have no debt in that regard. While I think it is morally right for university students retrospectively to pay back the debts incurred for their educational training, to give them a sense of responsibility and seriousness in their training, I find it dreadful that the necks of university graduates are saddled with debts they can never ever finish paying.

I am fully aware that there are different underlying factors limiting children from non-professional families in Zimbabwe, South Africa and the United Kingdom. In Zimbabwe we have missed a few corners and have forgotten the craft of social mobility. Zimbabwe started from scratch in creating a universal educational system that was not only robust and fit for purpose, but achieved the highest literacy rate in Africa within a blistering pace of ten years. Slowly but surely, we started extorting user fees from pupils and excluding the children who could not raise the money from attending school. I too was chased from Fletcher High School for non-payment of school fees. Many aspirations of children from poorer families vanished that way and there is an innumerable number of people in Zimbabwe who had an amputated educational path because of being unable to cough up the school fees. The practice has entrenched education and skills training to the wealthier Zimbabwean families. Probably the most effective way of investing in promising pupils in Zimbabwe from the non-professional families is to set up examination fee scholarships to A-level pupils, who have proven themselves during the O-levels. Examination fee scholarships are a smart way of avoiding high administrative costs of running the scholarships. Original hard copies of outstanding O-level certificates will have to be seen first and the money paid straight to the school of the highest ranked pupils. Further details on how to you can help by donating to the examination scholarships will be on the book website.[100]

South Africa has a different assortment of factors bedevilling and limiting social mobility of children from non-professional families. One of the things that has taken me aback is how very inefficient the educational institutions are in making children from non-professional families able to graduate from universities. South Africa has one of the lowest graduation rates in the whole world and only one out of every seven university students actually graduates (only 15% of the students graduate).[101] The problem has been taxing the minds of everyone in South Africa and there is no agreed consensus on what the

---

[100] www.youthaspirations.co.uk
[101] http://www.hsrc.ac.za/Document-2717.phtml

major problem is, let alone how to reduce the university dropout rate. I too honestly do not know how best to reduce the high dropout rate, especially of Africans in South Africa.

Britain, surprisingly, ranks very poorly among developed countries in terms of social mobility[102] and faces some peculiar challenges, which are different to those found in Zimbabwe. I am greatly touched by the huge upward social mobility that has occurred among the undergraduate African students that I taught in South Africa and Zimbabwe. It was the norm for virtually all of the graduates from the University of Zimbabwe to have a parent who had not gone to university. The greater bulk of Zimbabwean graduates from the medical school in Zimbabwe are now working as medical doctors, physiotherapists, nurses, occupational therapists and radiographers in Zimbabwe, neighbouring countries and abroad.

The ability to access and graduate from higher education is one of the core gears used to promote social mobility across the world. Britain has much to do in this regard and it has been noted that: *'the access to higher education, is at the heart of Britain's low mobility culture and what sets us apart from other European and North American countries.'* [103]

The picture of social mobility in Britain would be incomplete if the problem of undergraduate and postgraduate funding of children from poorer families is not considered. Most professional careers like accountancy, medicine, law, architecture and teaching require a postgraduate diploma or master's degree to get a full professional registration. Graduates wishing to pursue postgraduate studies have to brave taking a second loan

---

[102]http://www.guardian.co.uk/business/2010/mar/10/oecd-uk-worst-social-mobility
[103]http://www2.lse.ac.uk/newsAndMedia/news/archives/2005/LSE_SuttonTrust_repo rt.aspx and http://www.bis.gov.uk/assets/biscore/economics-and-statistics/docs/s/11-750-social-mobility-literature-review.pdf

from a bank, if they fail to get the competitive scholarships based on academic merit. The first loan (undergraduate student loan) will take the majority of new students 30 years to pay back at commercial interest rates. Graduates from poorer families might be very hesitant to then obtain a second loan and more likely to opt out of professional careers altogether.

The challenge of paddling upstream against seven 'fattened lions' to access the higher education and the above average hard work required to pass examinations may not be worth the hassle if the social security nets still guarantee a decent basic lifestyle. The government social security in Britain, which aims to provide benefits for vulnerable people in need, may inadvertently be depressing the future aspirations of young children from poorer families and restricting their future social mobility. I knew very well, even when I was still in primary school in Zimbabwe, that unless I took my future seriously, the vicious poverty cycle trap without social security, would continue for yet another generation. We knew the alternative all too well. This fostered a strong desire to achieve social mobility and a certain standard of living.

The financial advantages of working full time in Britain while on the minimum wage have failed to match the benefits of receiving social security and have trimmed the social mobility that develops from natural job promotion leading to career progression. The free associated services you get while on benefits, like free dental care, housing subsidies, travel and nursery day care concessions, vanish and they will be chargeable once you start working.[104] Another consideration affecting social mobility in Britain is the reduced tendency among lower paid young mothers to be employed. These fail to see the logic of

---

[104]http://www.unison.org.uk/acrobat/B1657.pdf- a polarized view of a workers union.

paying strangers to look after their children at a rate equivalent to the rate they are being paid. The mothers can care for their children with far more love, in the way they would like to and in a more bonding-conducive environment.

The ancient dilemmas of how to stop the social security safety nets from depressing work aspirations, having minimum wages that leave you worse off than being on state welfare, unemployed young mothers (who are often single) and how to tackle undergraduate funding, have heavily taxed the minds of society, politicians and economists. There are no easy answers to these complex and emotive issues.

This book is a call to all to be genuine, practical and relevant to our communities. Social networking websites like 'Twitter', 'Facebook' and blogs have gone viral because deep down people are longing for genuine messages from and interaction with authentic people. Personal reflection of our lives is far easier if we are honest and genuine. Genuineness will invariably have imperfection and hopefully we can learn a thing or two from the limitations of other people. I have been as open as day.

I have combed my past in a brutally frank manner, in the hope that I am being honest about the lives we have lived. I peeled the emotional onion life layers to expose doubts and my challenges. I would not ever wish any pupils to have a rough time and go through all my experiences, but I would like them to see what they can learn from it. Neither have I intended this account to be prescriptive or representative for any person who has gone through a scientific training. The book should rather be seen as a glimpse of how someone has handled sticky contemporary issues.

I have attempted to raise aspirations among children in the lower socioeconomic classes and do not look down on people doing menial or manual work. I would do any menial work if pushed by circumstances if that were the only way to pay my monthly bills. Moreover, I still have a lot of relatives and close friends who have been doing menial jobs for decades and who have helped me in one way or another as I was growing up. They have been great sources of emotional, financial and spiritual support along my educational journey.

The book had not been intended to be a lecture at all, but a simple narrative of convoluted and usual history. The lives we lead are never linear but are always convoluted in a multifactorial mesh. A bicycle puncture may occur on the day that you have misplaced your house keys while preparing for an assignment that is due the following morning. The same situation for a different person may be a breeze, while for someone else it could be the straw that breaks the camel's back.

The neighbourhoods and nicer friends we mingle with today will not always be around. It may seem rather ruthless to say so, but in ten years or so, you will be very unlikely to know the whereabouts of your current classmates. Neither is this book only advocating that a career in science is the only hallowed ground. The same dedication is sought after in other career fields.

Even if this whole project were to collapse, the very least it has done for me is to illuminate more clearly what God has done in my life. I have become more sensitive to those among us who are in similar shoes. The few people who have had a look at the book in its draft stages, such as relatives and friends, have remarked how the book has challenged their very lives. Some adults have felt that perhaps they should have obtained an extra qualification or two some time ago, while my mother is contemplating taking up distance learning for a university qualification at the age of 60 years.

The time is coming when you will apply for a degree programme and have to submit a motivational letter or 'personal statement'. You will have two options: either to describe how you gallantly battled against the 'fattened lions' or to be too ashamed to mention your social context and background. I would strongly urge you to note down your social, home and school contexts, as the ears of universities have become more receptive to disadvantaged students.[105] Universities in Britain are now systematically fast tracking and up-ranking applications of students from difficult social backgrounds and students from poor performing schools. The 'personal statement' will be an occasion to write a super condensed 'Educational Odyssey' of your life. Many a student has lost out on a university place because of not mentioning the social context in which their results were achieved.

Some of you who are reading this memoir may have underestimated the impact of your experiences or have lost the willpower to write it down. My desire is for adults to be more forthcoming in giving career advice to the young. School teachers and school administrators are in the best position to organise and invite other people to come and give career talks to the youth. Either way I hope my small autobiographical account of my brief life as a 34-year-old will spur you and inspire you to write, lest your life-changing memories vanish into thin air when you also leave. You might have far more years to draw lessons from or might have more tangible or illustrious days. The autobiography is a snapshot, or cross section, of a life channelled into a scientific career and it would be nice to read narratives that describe a life in the humanities or commerce as well. Perhaps God has given you a message of hope for us all!

---

[105]http://www.telegraph.co.uk/education/universityeducation/8799795/Universities-fast-tracking-poorer-students-Ucas-data-shows.html and http://www.universitiesuk.ac.uk/Publications/Documents/feti2.pdf

Chapter 20

Concluding Words

6 **I** N THE FUTURE YOUR CHILDREN will ask you, "What do these regulations, laws, and rules which the Lord our God commanded you mean to you?" Tell them, "We were Pharaoh's slaves in Egypt, but the Lord used his mighty hand to bring us out of there. Right before our eyes, the Lord did miraculous signs and amazing things that were spectacular but terrible for Egypt, Pharaoh, and his whole family. The Lord led us out of there to bring us here and give us this land he promised to our ancestors with an oath. The Lord our God commanded us to obey all these laws and to fear him. These laws are for our own good as long as we live so that He will preserve our lives. It is still true today. This is how we'll have the Lord's approval: If we faithfully obey all these laws in the presence of the Lord our God, as he has commanded us.'

Deuteronomy 6:20-25.

Lightning Source UK Ltd.
Milton Keynes UK
UKOW050240180412

190920UK00003B/3/P